WRITING COVID-19 LI

Writing COVID-19 Lives examines how people turned to life writing—often in fragile, makeshift forms—to make sense of the pandemic. Across poetry, memoir, autofiction, photography, sketchbooks, diaries, postcards, and digital storytelling, the collection traces a pandemic aesthetic marked by brevity, fracture, and pause: an autobiographical "I" that is unsettled, doubled, or dispersed. As Chimamanda Ngozi Adichie writes in *Notes on Grief*, "You learn how much grief is about language, the failure of language and the grasping for language." That grasping—the search for a voice that could still speak—threads through these essays.

Spanning case studies from Canada, the United States, China, Latvia, Peru, the United Kingdom, and Spain, the volume situates these works amid uneven conditions of care, precarity, surveillance, and loss. We encounter poetry written into silence; memoirs shaped by Zoom-mediated mourning; autofiction working through trauma; and photographic diaries—such as Marvin Heiferman's *Photographic Shiva*—that turn domestic objects into charged residues of grief.

Rather than offering a single story of "the pandemic," the volume assembles a textured archive of how lives were written—tenderly, urgently, and sometimes beautifully—under unprecedented constraint.

Irene Gammel, FRSC, is a professor of art, literature, and culture and the director of the Modern Literature and Culture (MLC) Centre at Toronto Metropolitan University. Her research explores life writing, trauma narratives, modern literature and visual culture, and the performance of self in public. She is the author and editor of 15 books, including *Looking for Anne of Green Gables: L.M. Montgomery and Her Timeless Heroine* (2025), *I Can Only Paint: The Story of Battlefield Artist Mary Riter Hamilton* (2020), and *Baroness Elsa: Gender, Dada and Everyday Modernity* (2002), and the winner of the C. P. Stacey Award. She has coedited many books including *Creative Resilience and COVID-19: Figuring the Everyday in a Pandemic* (Routledge, 2022). Her work investigates how individuals narrate personal and collective histories in times of crisis and cultural change.

Jason Wang's research explores how modernist and contemporary literature and media encode power, politics, and social values. His doctoral dissertation, entitled "Urban Walking: Configuring the Modern City as Cultural and Spatial Practice," explored the aesthetics of spatial politics and the politics of spatial aesthetics in urban literature and culture from the early twentieth century to the postindustrial period. He is the co-editor of *Creative Resilience and COVID-19: Figuring the Everyday in a Pandemic* (Routledge, 2022). He has contributed chapters to *Florine Stettheimer: New Directions in Multimodal Modernism* (2019) and *Confluences 2: Essays on the New Canadian Literature* (2017) as well as the *Routledge Encyclopedia of Modernism*. Wang is a lecturer at Toronto Metropolitan University's School of Fashion.

The COVID-19 Pandemic Series

Series Editor: J. Michael Ryan

This series examines the impact of the COVID-19 pandemic on individuals, communities, countries, and the larger global society from a social scientific perspective. It represents a timely and critical advance in knowledge related to what many believe to be the greatest threat to global ways of being in more than a century. It is imperative that academics take their rightful place alongside medical professionals as the world attempts to figure out how to deal with the current global pandemic, and how society might move forward in the future. This series represents a response to that imperative.

Titles in this Series:

Viral World
Global Relations During the COVID-19 Pandemic
Long T. Bui

Folk Devils and Moral Panics in the COVID-19 Pandemic
Edited by Morena Tartari, Cosimo Marco Scarcelli and Cirus Rinaldi

Moral Panics and Social Control in the Covid-19 Pandemic
Edited by Morena Tartari, Cirus Rinaldi and Riccardo Caldarera

Writing COVID-19 Lives
Edited by Irene Gammel and Jason Wang

For more information about this series, please visit:
https://www.routledge.com/The-COVID-19-Pandemic-Series/book-series/CVIDPAN

WRITING COVID-19 LIVES

Edited by Irene Gammel and Jason Wang

Routledge
Taylor & Francis Group
LONDON AND NEW YORK

Designed cover image: Excerpt from the Pandemic Diary of Anna Meiere Logina ID 166-77-5, Latvian Pandemic Diary Collection.

First published 2026
by Routledge
4 Park Square, Milton Park, Abingdon, Oxon OX14 4RN

and by Routledge
605 Third Avenue, New York, NY 10158

Routledge is an imprint of the Taylor & Francis Group, an informa business

British Library Cataloguing-in-Publication Data
A catalogue record for this book is available from the British Library

ISBN: 978-1-041-23153-0 (hbk)
ISBN: 978-1-041-23154-7 (pbk)
ISBN: 978-1-003-73559-5 (ebk)

DOI: 10.4324/9781003735595

Typeset in Times New Roman
by Apex CoVantage, LLC

CONTENTS

FIGURES

CONTRIBUTORS

Kristina Bhaun is a doctoral student of communication and culture at Toronto Metropolitan University (TMU) and a doctoral research fellow at the Modern Literature and Culture Research Centre, where she contributes to the *Telling COVID-19 Stories* digital project. Her research focuses on the intersection of archives, preservation, and COVID-19 stories. She holds an MA in literatures of modernity from Toronto Metropolitan University and a BA in English with minors in the history and philosophy of science and in French from the University of Toronto.

Marjorie Dryburgh is a lecturer in modern Chinese studies at the School of East Asian Studies, University of Sheffield. Dryburgh works on memory, life story, and regional social histories of China, with specific interests in childhood and family story and the interplay between personal and collective registers of history. She is the co-editor of *Writing Lives in China, 1600–2010: Histories of the Elusive Self* (Palgrave, 2013). Her scholarly work was published in various journals, including "My Manchuria: Memoir, Manga, and the Legacies of Japanese Wartime Childhoods" in *The Journal of the History of Childhood and Youth* (2023); "Life Histories and National Narratives: Remembering Occupied Manchuria in Postwar China" in *History Workshop Journal* (2019); and "Re-centering Education in Manshūkoku (1931–1945): School and Family in Chinese Oral History" in *Japan Forum* (2019).

Irene Gammel, FRSC, is a professor of art, literature, and culture and the director of the Modern Literature and Culture (MLC) Centre at Toronto Metropolitan University. Her research explores life writing, trauma narratives, modern literature and visual culture, and the performance of self in public. She is the author and editor of 15 books, including *Looking for Anne of Green Gables: L.M. Montgomery and Her*

Timeless Heroine (Sutherland House Books, 2025), *I Can Only Paint: The Story of Battlefield Artist Mary Riter Hamilton* (McGill-Queen's University Press, 2020), and *Baroness Elsa: Gender, Dada and Everyday Modernity* (MIT Press, 2002), and the winner of the C. P. Stacey Award. She has coedited many books including *Creative Resilience and COVID-19: Figuring the Everyday in a Pandemic* (Routledge, 2022). Her work investigates how individuals narrate personal and collective histories in times of crisis and cultural change.

Ana Belén Martínez García is an associate professor of English at the University of Navarra, Spain, and collaborates with the Bonds, Creativity and Culture hub (VCC) at the Institute for Culture and Society (ICS). She is part of the research project "Re-orienting Assemblage Theory in Anglophone Literature and Culture" and "RELY" and co-leads WG5 "Human Stories for Humane Reactions." Her research focuses on human rights testimonies by young and displaced activists and how narrative empathy works online and offline. Her publications have been featured in journals such as *a/b: Auto/Biography Studies*, *Life Writing*, *Prose Studies*, and *Narrative*. She is the author of *New Forms of Self-Narration: Young Women, Life Writing and Human Rights* (Palgrave, 2020) and has co-edited *Representing 21st-Century Migration in Europe: Performing Borders, Identities and Texts* (Berghahn, 2022).

Christopher J. Gilbert is a professor of English at Assumption University, Massachusetts, whose research explores the intersection of humor, culture, and politics, particularly how public communication reflects and influences societal values during periods of conflict. His books include *When Comedy Goes Wrong* (Indiana University Press, 2025) and *Caricature and National Character: The United States at War* (Penn State University Press, 2021). Gilbert is also the co-editor of *Pleasure and Pain in US Public Culture* (University of Alabama Press, 2024) and associate editor for *Studies in American Humor*. His work has appeared in journals such as *Quarterly Journal of Speech* and *Studies in American Humor*, with notable articles like "The Diapered Donald: Comic Infantilizations of a U.S. American President" (2021).

Ilze Ļaksa-Timinska is a researcher at the Institute of Literature, Folklore and Art, University of Latvia, where she specializes in life writing, Soviet-era literary culture, and cultural history. She oversees the Autobiography Collection at the Archives of Latvian Folklore and has played a leading role in curating the Latvian Pandemic Diary project. Her work foregrounds marginalized literary voices and the role of personal narrative in collective memory, and she has been recognized with the Young Scientist Prize by the Latvian Academy of Sciences. Her recent publications address the intersections of ideology and folklore and the potential of digital platforms to support citizen science in the humanities.

Brent Luvaas is a professor of global studies and a graduate faculty member at Communication, Culture, & Media, Drexel University. A visual and cultural anthropologist, his work explores how digital technologies shape the way we see and experience the world around us. He is the author of *Street Style: An Ethnography of Fashion Blogging* (Bloomsbury, 2016) and *DIY Style: Fashion, Music, and Global Digital Cultures* (Berg, 2012). His book *Street Style* was the 2019 winner of the John Collier Jr. Award for Still Photography.

Haralds Matulis is a research assistant at the Institute of Literature, Folklore and Art, University of Latvia, and a doctoral student at the Faculty of Humanities at the same institution. Trained in philosophy, anthropology, and literary studies, he focuses on computational and digital methodologies in the humanities, particularly in relation to archival and autobiographical corpora. Matulis has contributed to several research projects on metadata modeling, diary analysis, and text corpora creation, with recent work exploring automated date detection and corpus linguistics for underrepresented Latvian literary voices. His interdisciplinary approach bridges traditional literary analysis and digital tools.

Julie Rak (FRSC) is a professor and H.M. Tory chair at the Department of English and Film Studies, the University of Alberta, Canada. Her books include *False Summit: Gender in Mountaineering Nonfiction* (McGill-Queen's University Press, 2021), *Boom! Manufacturing Memoir for the Popular Market* (Wilfrid Laurier University Press, 2013), and *Negotiated Memory: Doukhobor Autobiographical Discourse* (University of British Columbia Press, 2004). She is the editor of the *Identities* volume of the *Oxford Encyclopedia of Literary Theory* (2021) and the collection *Autobiography in Canada* (2005). She has co-edited *Identity Technologies: Constructing the Self Online* (University of Wisconsin Press, 2014). She co-edited the reissue of Inuk author Mini Aodla Freeman's memoir, *Life Among the Qallunaat* (University of Manitoba Press, 2014), Philippe Lejeune's *On Diary* (University of Hawaii Press, 2009), and *Mountain Masculinity: The Writings of Nello "Tex" Vernon-Wood, 1911–1938* (Athabasca University Press, 2008). Her latest book is *The Routledge Introduction to Auto/biography in Canada* (Taylor & Francis, 2022), co-written with Sonja Boon, Laurie McNeill, and Candida Rifkind. She holds an SSHRC IDG grant on contemporary journaling as a post-digital practice.

Sanita Reinsone is an associate professor at the Digital Humanities Center, University of Latvia, where her research focuses on participatory heritage, digital archiving, and life writing. She has led numerous national and international projects, including pioneering work in crowdsourced cultural heritage and digital life story collections. Her publications span theoretical and applied approaches to digital humanities and include *The Poetics of Getting Lost in Legends, Stories,* *and Conversations* (LU LFMI, 2017, in Latvian), as well as documentary books such as *Forest Daughters* (Dienas Grāmata, 2015) and *Story of Ādams* (Zinātne, 2008), both adapted for the stage. Reinsone's recent work, including in the *European Journal of Life Writing* and Routledge collections, explores the ethical and methodological complexities of documenting everyday experiences through collaborative digital means.

J. Michael Ryan is a professor of sociology at the Pontificia Universidad Católica del Perú and an editor specializing in gender, sexuality, and social policy. His research explores sociocultural dimensions of COVID-19 and the intersectional experiences of marginalized communities. He is the author, with Serena Nanda, of *COVID-19: Social Inequalities and Human Possibilities* (Routledge, 2022) and co-editor of over 15 volumes, including *COVID-19: Global Pandemic, Societal Responses, Ideological Solutions* (Routledge, 2021) and *Core Concepts in Sociology* (Wiley, 2019). Ryan is also the founding editor of Routledge's *The COVID-19 Pandemic* book series.

Jason Wang's research explores how modernist and contemporary literature and media encode power, politics, and social values. His doctoral dissertation, entitled "Urban Walking: Configuring the Modern City as Cultural and Spatial Practice," explored the aesthetics of spatial politics and the politics of spatial aesthetics in urban literature and culture from the early twentieth century to the postindustrial period. He is the co-editor of *Creative Resilience and COVID-19: Figuring the Everyday in a Pandemic* (Routledge, 2022). He has contributed chapters to *Florine Stettheimer: New Directions in Multimodal Modernism* (Book*hug Press, 2019) and *Confluences 2: Essays on the New Canadian Literature* (Mawenzi House, 2017) as well as the *Routledge Encyclopedia of Modernism*. Wang is a lecturer at Toronto Metropolitan University's School of Fashion.

Julia Watson is an academy professor emerita of comparative studies at The Ohio State University. A leading scholar in life narrative studies, she specializes in feminist theory, women's writing, graphic memoir, and postcolonial life writing. With Sidonie Smith, she co-authored the influential *Reading Autobiography: A Guide for Interpreting Life Narratives* (2nd expanded ed., 2010) and co-edited five foundational volumes, including *Before They Could Vote: American Women's Autobiographical Writing, 1819–1919* (2006) and *De/Colonizing the Subject: The Politics of Gender in Women's Autobiography* (1992). Their collected essays, *Life Writing in the Long Run: A Smith & Watson Autobiography Studies Reader* (2017), are available in open-access format. Watson's recent work includes the essay "Days of Reckoning: Prospects for Live Narrative—2020" in *The Untied States: Unraveling National Identities in the Twenty-First Century* (2021) and "Drawing Is the Best Medicine: Somatic Dis-ease and Graphic Revenge in Miriam Katin's *Letting It Go*" (*Biography*, Autumn 2021). Her work continues to shape the field of life writing in times of personal and political reckoning.

Marjorie Worthington is a professor of English and women's, gender, and sexuality studies at Eastern Illinois University, where she specializes in contemporary American literature and experimental fiction. Her scholarly contributions have appeared in journals such as *Critique*, *Studies in the Novel*, *Genre*, *LIT: Literature, Interpretation, Theory*, *Papers on Language and Literature*, and *Twentieth-Century Literature*. Worthington's book, *The Story of "Me": Contemporary American Autofiction*, was published by the University of Nebraska Press in 2018.

Elvīra Žvarte is a research assistant at the Institute of Literature, Folklore and Art, University of Latvia and a PhD candidate at the Latvian Academy of Culture. With a background in social anthropology, her research centers on life writing, memory work, and collaborative autobiographical practices, particularly among older adults. She has contributed to major projects involving digital archiving and editorial work within the Autobiography Collection and the Digital Archives of Latvian Folklore. Žvarte's scholarship engages with the ethics and aesthetics of documenting lived experience, often foregrounding community-based approaches to narrative and memory in contemporary Latvian culture.

ACKNOWLEDGMENTS

Editing *Writing COVID-19 Lives* has been both a privilege and a responsibility. This volume gathers voices that dared to speak, write, and experiment in the midst of rupture, with many contributors inspired by their own personal diaries and expressions—even visual expressions. All chapters are original and exclusive to this volume. The book has benefited from our *Telling COVID-19 Stories Digital Databank*, launched in 2024.

We acknowledge, first, the courage of our contributors, who entrusted us with essays that bear witness to individual and collective experiences during this time of crisis. Their words remind us that even in isolation, we were never alone.

A volume of essays is a collective undertaking shaped not only by the scholarship, creativity, and critical insight of its contributors but also by the groundwork that made such a project possible. This book would not exist without the team support of the Modern Literature and Culture (MLC) Research Centre—including research assistants Enya Jovicik and Cigdem Asatekin MacInnis, and MLC coordinator Ella Altena—whose steady attention to detail, help with coordination, and day-to-day support helped sustain the editorial process over many months.

Routledge's Pandemic Series Editor, J. Michael Ryan, championed this project from its initial proposal to final production, and his steady involvement helped anchor the book at key stages. Senior Editor Alice Salt guided its development, including the decision to publish both hardcover and paperback editions, ensuring that the book reaches readers inside and outside academia. The Routledge editorial and production team—from copyeditor to designer—brought a level of care that shaped not only the readability of the text but also the accessibility of the volume as a tool meant to be used, not merely shelved.

This study benefited from financial support from the Social Sciences and Humanities Research Council of Canada; the Canada Foundation for Innovation;

and the Ontario Ministry of Research, Innovation and Science, which provided infrastructure funds to the Modern Literature and Culture Research Centre; as well as the Office of the Vice-President, Research and Innovation, the Provost's Office, and the Dean of Arts Office at Toronto Metropolitan University.

Thank you, all.

The Editors
Modern Literature and Culture Research Centre
Toronto Metropolitan University mlc.torontomu.ca

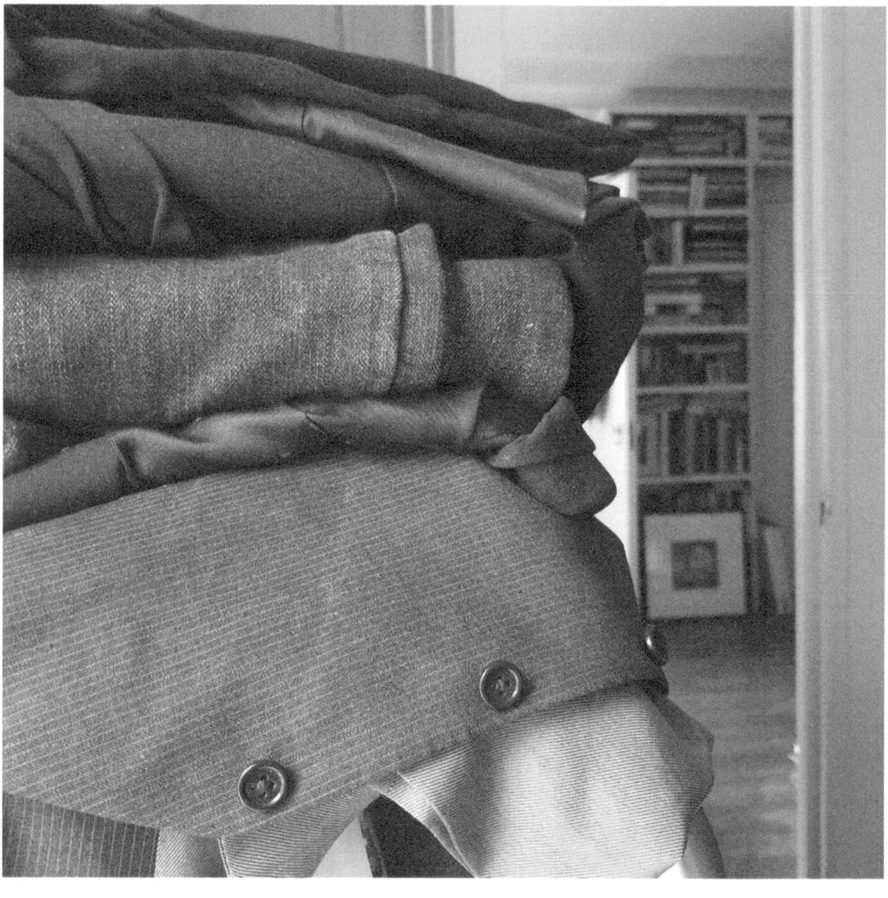

FIGURE 0.0 Marvin Heiferman, "A pile of Maurice's everyday, wear-around-the-house clothes that I've yet to deal with . . ." Photograph posted on Instagram, whywelook, 10 April 2022. https://www.instagram.com/p/CcLzM2guXNm/.

INTRODUCTION

Writing COVID-19 Lives

Irene Gammel and Jason Wang

"For weeks, my stomach is in turmoil, tense and tight with foreboding, the ever-present certainty that somebody else will die, that more will be lost." In *Notes on Grief* (2021), Chimamanda Ngozi Adichie writes about the aftermath of the death of her father during the COVID-19 pandemic, her memoir becoming a stark reflection on the challenges of mourning in a time when even grief was Zoom-mediated—when the rituals of loss were fragmented and refracted through screens. As Adichie writes, "You learn how much grief is about language, the failure of language and the grasping for language."[1] The second person "you" operates not as an address to the reader but as a displaced "I," signaling a fractured interiority. In moments of emotional rupture, the self becomes unmoored from its narrative anchor, speaking to itself in the guise of another.

This I–you dynamic, an internal doubling, captures the dissociative logic of pandemic life writing, where subjectivity is not only narrated but also dispersed, estranged and in the process of reassembly.

Another deeply touching self-narrative, this one in photography, is Marvin Heiferman's "Photographic Shiva"—a self-portrait series created after his partner died of COVID-19. Posted on his Instagram account, one image—featured here as the frontispiece (Figure 0.0)—shows a pile of folded clothing: pants, a purple shirt, blue jeans, a vest with its buttons undone and aligned horizontally, the opposite of the live, vertical position, outside an empty room. The clothing dominates the immediate foreground, occupying two-thirds of the vertical frame, overwhelming the viewer. In the background, the rest of the apartment sits empty: a bookcase, the open door to a vacant room. As a self-portrait, this threshold space of mourning is charged with affect—the desire to hold onto a loved one's memory, to honor a relationship that has ended—and the sense of being overwhelmed by the process. In the Instagram posting, Heiferman's caption reads: "A pile of Maurice's everyday,

DOI: 10.4324/9781003735595-1

wear-around-the-house clothes that I've yet to deal with . . . ."[2] The slow work of mourning—still in process—finds expression in this form of visual diary shared with a community of Instagram followers who sympathize, "You don't need to deal with them till you want to," the painter Ilona Anderson replies.[3] In another photograph from Heiferman's series, two wedding rings appear side by side, no longer worn, quietly marking absence in this diary of mourning, creating stories which this volume of essays seeks to unpack. Heiferman's images, like so many pandemic self-narratives, illustrate that life writing during COVID-19 often blurred boundaries between the personal and the public, the visual and the verbal, the intimate and the shared. This impulse—to process, to witness, to connect—animates the essays that follow this introduction.

In this volume, we present ten essays and a coda that examine how life writing practices emerged, shifted, and were redefined in response to the COVID-19 pandemic across varied cultural, social, and geographical contexts. It brings together case studies that consider not only what individuals wrote about their lives under pandemic conditions but also how and why they wrote. At its core, this collection understands life writing during the pandemic not simply as a form of testimony or documentation, but as a mode of sense-making—reconfiguring subjectivity, community, and politics through the constraints and affordances of crisis. The pandemic has accelerated an ongoing transformation in life writing studies, which has long moved beyond coherent, retrospective self-narratives toward fractured, collective, and multimodal forms of self-representation. We take up and extend Sidonie Smith and Julia Watson's theorization of life writing or life narratives as diverse kinds of life stories and practices of telling one's life in different forms, textual, visual, and performative. Thus, they think of self-representational work less in terms of "autobiography" than "as enacted life narratives."[4] Across these chapters, contributors engage with diverse media—postcards, diaries, poetry, memoir, sketches, photographs—to show that pandemic life writing often foregrounded process over product, provisionality over polish, and interruption over resolution. These aesthetic choices are not merely stylistic; they emerge from and respond to the emotional dislocations of the pandemic—fear, grief, boredom—as well as the structural limitations that shaped expression: censorship, precarity, inequality, and enforced isolation. These works suggest that form itself became a site where the pandemic's lived contradictions were registered and negotiated.

Underpinning this volume is the recognition that the pandemic exposed how unevenly the capacity to narrate one's life is distributed across the globe. Life writing, long assumed to be an individual, literate, and often privileged act, became during COVID-19 a register of structural inequality: who could isolate safely, who could speak publicly, who could mourn aloud. By reading pandemic narratives through this lens, the essays collected here engage with life writing not as a universal human practice but as a socially contingent and politically charged one. From digital self-portraits circulating in the Global North to collective diary projects in Latvia and testimonies of refugees, the chapters reveal that the power to tell one's story is inseparable from the material conditions of survival. In foregrounding these disparities, the volume frames pandemic life writing as an ethical field—one that measures not only what was written but also what could not be.

The volume develops along three key methodological trajectories. First, this volume foregrounds life writing's capaciousness for *self-exploration during the pandemic*, while also considering the relational and contingent nature of pandemic self-writing—that is, how life writers' expressions of self are shaped by specific conditions such as their social position, emotional experience, digital connectivity, and cultural context. Across the contributions, life writing is understood as a mode of entanglement—with others, with publics, with platforms, with structures of power. In the first section, Julia Watson descends into the past, into memory work, using COVID-19 to reflect on how earlier experiences of illness, caregiving, and loss resurface under the strain of pandemic time. In our own essay, Irene Gammel and Jason Wang look at the use of gaps and silences as a life writing strategy during COVID-19, examining the surge of poetry during the pandemic, while Marjorie Worthington considers autofiction's role in working through the aftershocks, whereby COVID-19 autofiction becomes a trauma narrative. Similarly, Marjorie Dryburgh's analysis of Chinese COVID-19 diaries reveals how self-narration operated in tension with surveillance and censorship, calling into question what kinds of autobiographical agency were available in highly restrictive social and political contexts.

Second, it emphasizes life writing as an archival method—spanning personal records, collective initiatives, and institutionally supported projects. These practices challenge normative assumptions about whose stories—and lives—are preserved, how they are told, and what forms are valued. They include vernacular modes that emerge from everyday habits or digital platforms, as well as feminist interventions within formal archives. In their essay on the Sheffield Feminist Archive's postcard project, Kristina Bhaun and Irene Gammel explore women's empowerment through the inscription of pandemic experiences in non-normative forms. These creative acts resist dominant narratives and the erasure of gendered care work, illness, and grief. Such archives function not only as sites of memory but also as critical interventions into what is recognized as historically significant during times of crisis.

Sanita Reinsone and her co-authors examine Latvia's crowdsourced Pandemic Diary Collection, launched in March 2020 to gather personal accounts of life under COVID-19. While the project reveals how life writing can shape collective memory in crisis, the chapter also exposes tensions around trauma, representation, and the limits of rapid-response archiving. As Julie Rak notes, self-narration is shaped by structures of solicitation, revealing how stories are drawn out, framed, and made legible. Life writing thus functions as a political method, creating an ethics of witnessing rooted in everyday practices, partial perspectives, and resistant care.

Third, the volume examines how *the pandemic reshaped media ecologies*, altering not only daily life but also the ways it was documented, mediated, and understood. Ana Belén Martínez García analyzes Syrian political refugee Hassan Akkad's digital storytelling—his viral 2020 NHS scrubs video helped change UK policy—and shows how his memoir extends this digital voice into literary form, using care and assemblage theories to trace trauma's collective impact. Brent Luvaas turns ethnographic attention inward through photography, capturing domestic spaces as sites of emotional and spatial experience during lockdown, revealing how interior life became a rich terrain for visual life writing. Christopher J. Gilbert's daily sketches and written reflections explore informal, visual self-representation as a private, affective coping strategy, highlighting how life writing can function meaningfully without an expected audience. Together, as J. Michael Ryan's Coda shows, these chapters explore life writing's evolving forms during COVID-19, emphasizing its relational, experimental, and collective dimensions despite disrupted media infrastructures.

Underpinning this collection of essays is the belief that life writing is inherently political: personal narratives can contest dominant histories, expose structures of inequality, and assert the value of marginalized experience. In some chapters, life writing becomes a powerful tool for addressing issues of forced migration, labor, and racialized identities, linking the personal with collective struggles and exposing the socio-political implications of these experiences. Similarly, other essays underscore how grief and personal memory can resonate within broader public crises, where the boundaries between private suffering and collective trauma blur, drawing attention to the political dimensions of social isolation. Still other chapters explore processes of normalization as contested terrains where seemingly ordinary acts—like remembrance, silence, or everyday storytelling—become sites of both complicity and resistance, exposing how power operates through the subtle shaping of identity and memory. These examples show that life writing is not merely a personal exercise but a dynamic, political space for amplifying voices working within and beyond established structures, challenging entrenched power structures and reframes individual experiences in the context of broader social and political realities.

Theoretically, the volume draws from a range of cross-disciplinary traditions—including poststructuralist philosophy (e.g., Derrida's notion of the postcard and the instability of communication), feminist archival theory, trauma studies, visual anthropology, autoethnography, and digital life writing scholarship—to interrogate how the pandemic unsettled established norms of authorship, audience, justice, truth, and temporality. Coming from diverse fields across the arts, humanities, and social sciences, all contributions are grounded in life writing studies, particularly the frameworks developed by Philippe Lejeune, Paul John Eakin, Sidonie Smith, and Julia Watson, which provide a critical lens for examining the construction of self-narration under crisis, offering methodologically pluralistic yet thematically cohesive accounts. Several essays take up the notion of *disrupted time*: the ways in which lockdown and illness shattered conventional chronologies, leading to narratives that are episodic, recursive, or fragmented.

Others interrogate the unstable positioning of the autobiographical "I," which often appears dispersed, relational, or performative—shaped by the conditions of digital surveillance, platformed visibility, and collective mourning.

As a whole, the chapters in *Writing COVID-19 Lives* chart a critical genealogy of pandemic self-representation. They offer insight not only into the pandemic as an event but also into the future of life writing studies. What kinds of stories can be told under conditions of disruption? Whose stories get recorded, archived, and amplified—and whose are silenced or lost? How do everyday texts—postcards, poems, sketches, diaries—expand the boundaries of autobiography? By addressing these questions, this volume offers a grounded, theoretically engaged, socially and creatively attuned intervention into the field.

The contributors to this volume are primarily educators and researchers, writing from both the centers and the margins of cultural and institutional representation. Their lived experiences complicate and, at times, contest dominant narratives of the COVID-19 pandemic, expanding the critical and geographical reach of life writing scholarship. Representing diverse epicenters across four continents—including Canada, the United States, China, Latvia, Peru, the United Kingdom, and Spain—the volume reflects a spectrum of pandemic experiences, revealing both unexpected points of convergence and significant divergence. What unites these contributors is a shared commitment to rendering the lived experience of the COVID-19 pandemic through first-person, nonfictional narrative and scholarly reflection. While designed for use in the university classroom and cross-disciplinary research communities studying the COVID-19 pandemic, the volume is written in an accessible style for broader audiences interested in life writing, memoir, diary, archival studies, medical humanities, trauma studies, public health humanities, and narrative medicine. We also hope it will serve readers concerned with questions of affect, embodiment, and the documentation of crisis as a valuable resource for understanding the multiple contours of COVID-19 lives.

This volume builds on the groundwork laid in our previous book, *Creative Resilience and COVID-19: Figuring the Everyday in a Pandemic* (Routledge, 2022), which examines how individuals and communities navigated the early months of the global crisis through acts of creativity and reflection. That collection approached the pandemic through an understanding of crisis space and time, showing how the experience enforced a reconceptualization of everyday life—changes that have had lasting impact. In addition, our collaborative essay, "Taking Responsibility: COVID-19 and the Possibilities for Participatory Communication During Crisis," in the volume of *COVID-19: Individual Rights and Community Responsibilities* (2023), further explored how our research center pivoted in March 2020 to become a platform for COVID-19 communication, ultimately curating the longest-running COVID-19 webinar exchange in North America. We conceived of these gatherings in the spirit of the salons—intimate, reflective, and improvisational—with participants joining from bedrooms, kitchens, and basement offices.

Similarly, contributors to this volume invite readers into their personal spaces, intimate experiences, and everyday negotiations of the pandemic. These projects converge here in a collective inquiry the pandemic as a life writing moment, one that prompted a surge of diaries, letters, essays, and creative practices that document the disrupted textures of daily life. What explains this pronounced drive toward self-narration during COVID-19, especially when such impulses were largely absent during the 1918–19 influenza pandemic? What other questions of voice, witnessing, and cultural memory emerge as central to pandemic-era storytelling? This volume of essays addresses these questions.

Notes

1 Chimamanda Ngozi Adichie, *Notes on Grief: A Memoir* (Knopf, 2021), 6.
2 Marvin Heiferman, "A Pile of Maurice's Everyday, Wear-Around-the-House Clothes That I've yet to Deal with . . .," Photograph Posted on Instagram, whywelook, April 10, 2022, https://www.instagram.com/p/CcLzM2guXNm/.
3 Ilona Anderson, Post on Instagram, ilonapainter, April 10, 2022, https://www.instagram.com/p/CcLzM2guXNm/.
4 Sidonie Smith and Julia Watson, "Introduction," In *Interfaces: Women, Autobiography, Image, Performance* (University of Michigan Press, 2002), 8–9.

PART I

Life Writing as Pandemic Self-Exploration

1

WHAT IS A PANDEMIC GOOD FOR? BLURRED DAYS AND LIVE MEMORIES

Julia Watson

What is a pandemic good for? The losses have been grievous and massive, especially in the United States. Yet for some, the forced stillness brought an unsettling relief. When life ground to a halt in March 2020, I was stunned but also secretly grateful. Freed from the pressures of constant obligations, I could cast off both the detritus of past years and the weight of future plans. No trips to Michigan, Savannah, or Europe. Just the here and now. Though I had retired almost six years earlier, I remained immersed in writing, emails, and conferences—the most pleasurable aspects of my academic career. Yet I'd begun to wonder what it would feel like to live day by day, untethered from goals and deadlines. A small thought lingered: I needed time to catch up to the present, to confront the strange sense of being suspended between past and future.

Also, how do you frame a pandemic that's gutting the whole world? As a humanist, I was trained to approach crises from multiple perspectives—historical, political, aesthetic, and personal. COVID-19 tested those frameworks. In *The New York Times* (June 2020), graphic memoirist Alison Bechdel noted a strange calm amid the devastation, observing, "Some sort of deep transformational change is afoot inside of me, as it is in all of us."[1] Her words struck a chord. If grief and fear defined the pandemic's external reality, its inner currents were attuned to the workings of memory, narrative, and self-understanding. For me, the pandemic became not only a rupture but also a space for reflection and reckoning in journal form.

As I read this journal in 2025, the pandemic seems long ago and far away, though I still get vaccines against COVID and carry a mask. Rereading my "Covidious Chronicles," some published here, casts me back to that strange, melancholic time when many feared this unknown disease and wondered whether we and our loved ones would survive it. (And we all know someone who didn't.) The solitude

DOI: 10.4324/9781003735595-3

of days made it oddly like living in an earlier century, though we relied on virtual technologies and media like never before.

When I was asked to write an introduction for my chronicles on the contemporary memoirs I turned to during the pandemic, I was stymied. I didn't in fact reread narratives such as Joan Didion's *The Year of Magical Thinking* (2005). Yes, I thought about plague literature, particularly Boccaccio's *Decameron* (1353), which I hadn't read since grad school days; but its world of charmed storytelling was far from my homebound experience. I often recalled the worlds of uneasy tension and isolation in Albert Camus's *The Plague* (1947) and Thomas Mann's *Death in Venice* (1912). But stories of The Before Time didn't fit—I wanted immediacy, reports from the front. Graphic memoirists, working with the documentary power of images, were more compelling. Alison Bechdel's cartoons captured how "all the days really are blurring into one another."[2] Lynda Barry's terrific pandemic diary project took up "documenting all the small things that are easily lost."[3] And writer Leslie Jamison's exploration of how her life was reshaped "when the world went away" resonated with my own experience.[4]

I also took to reading obituaries, which the *New York Times* regularly published on the deaths from COVID of both famous and ordinary people. One of the first to die from its complications, on 7 April 2020, was singer/songwriter John Prine, a true "diamond in the rough."[5] But there could be no concert to mourn him collectively. Like many of us, I was stunned by the struggles of healthcare and essential workers and the terrible isolation of senior citizens in nursing homes. Although the jagged rhythm of slow days was punctuated by outbursts of police violence and demonstrations against racism, like Leslie Jamison, at home I was finding "an unexpected abundance inside a state of loss."[6]

The life narrative I read during the pandemic that continued to haunt my thinking was Tove Ditlevsen's *The Copenhagen Trilogy*: *Childhood-Youth-Dependency* (1967–71), a Danish memoir trilogy of the mid-twentieth century. It is the darkest work I've read in years and its merciless candor and clarity are truly "awful but joyful," as Deborah Eisenberg's incisive review declared.[7] Ditlevsen's terse narration of her bleak working-class childhood, menial jobs, and relentless adult use of opiates is tough but never self-pitying. It became a kind of character armament for getting through pandemic days.

Sidonie Smith, my co-author for *Reading Autobiography Now* (2024), and I were, as usual, at work on a project. This time it was an essay for a collection on American life narratives about navigating our fractured country, *The Divided States* (2023), edited by two astute autobiography scholars, Laura Beard and Ricia Chansky. In it we link autobiographical reckonings—when "one is called to account for one's actions"—to the disturbing, precarious pandemic days of 2020, haunted by the murder of George Floyd and others that reignited the Black Lives Matter movement in the United States.[8]

An essay note hints at what became my obsessive interest in mortality during that time. It concerns the Death Cafés on Zoom, "death-positive" gatherings of strangers who tell personal stories of how mortality affects the living. These *café mortel* events are a twenty-first-century phenomenon, inspired by the Swiss sociologist Bernard Crettaz who started one in 2004, and the British web designer Jon Underwood, who developed the model and convened a Death Café at his London home in 2011. At such gatherings, the "death-curious" were invited to tell stories across ages, genders, and races and to return to practices of family care centered on dying in earlier centuries. Although participation in death cafés was virtual on websites such as Deathcafe.com, they signaled a collective desire to revive rituals of communal mourning.[9] That resonated.

When COVID slammed into American awareness in March 2020, it exerted a compelling force on daily life. Now, we live mostly in The After Time, which may contribute to collective amnesia about the bodily sensations and anxieties stirred up by the pandemic. As a piece of memory work, I offer these fragments drawn from experiences of how it felt to be living then.

April 2020: The Dead-Letter Box

One of the peculiar and little-mentioned aspects of online communication is how people just slip out of your life without notice. You send them emails and never hear back. Was it something I said? Or has something happened to you? It's unnerving, not least because one's sadness is deferred for months or even years.

And sometimes, something really has happened. Somebody has died, and you just don't find out. People are dispersed all over this global world. So many of us live alone that there's no one to make the connection, call the relatives, write the obituary, and send a form reply to all the unanswered email. It's remarkable that no one has thought about how to address this. What about some kind of single button that you push on the computer when the end is nigh, like the nuclear button on the presidential red phone?

In this COVID time, such thoughts no longer seem too dark or socially unutterable. No, they're practical considerations—before someone slips away, before the ambulance comes and the intubation starts, just a warning note that they might not be returning. We won't be there in person—no one can be, anyway—but it would be consoling, if it comes to that. Like a status update.

A haunting question concerns grief. How can we grieve those who may have been lost at a distance? Friends, relatives, or colleagues who die alone, in an ICU where those close to them cannot be present to hold a hand, smooth a forehead, whisper words of love and gratitude that might get past the fog of coma. It is a cruel and heartless situation, if necessarily so.

I have not personally lost anyone I know to COVID—yet. Half of my 12 cousins are older than I, and some are fragile. The same is true for friends, and their partners. I find myself repeatedly asking after them. But worry is not a rational emotion. Or, in these times, maybe it is. We are discovering that we are all fragile. It is one of the lessons nature is imposing, in its own fragility and its relentless indifference. It seems that loss is a central lesson of life. Or, simply, a fact. In my younger, live-forever years, this truth was not so obvious. Now, it will inform the experience of even our children and grandchildren. Darwinism refurbished for our times.

Last year I lost three people, all close to me, all cherished. It was pre-COVID, but with similar issues. The first was my much younger, only sister. After being diminished by serious illness she seemed stable, but over two days, she suddenly up and died. I could not be there, nor was there a funeral or graveside/crematorium ritual. Just the pain of sudden, shocking loss. The "celebration of her life" six weeks later, in the Utah countryside, was large and sumptuous, with groaning tables of food from her dozens of chef-friends. Despite Motown playing nonstop, it was the least celebratory event I've ever attended. Though tears flowed everywhere, I would have preferred an Irish wake with cursing and wailing.

The second person was my high school would-be boyfriend Jim, whom I'd later grown close to: letters sent from and to Vietnam during the war, a SoCal fling when we both lived there, reconnection when on impulse I sent him a Christmas greeting in 2009. He lived in deepest Texas, was an alcoholic with five children, on his third wife—a Mexican immigrant half his age—and a "libertarian." With the tempering of age and the pleasure of memories, we developed a frequently hilarious correspondence about everything from sports to family to philosophical questions. And we had some wonderfully romantic meet-ups here and there. Even though we feuded in the fall of 2016, on the eve of the election, when he emailed that he was tired of my "elite liberal bullshit"—I knew that code—we stayed in occasional and affectionate contact. Jim was getting his shopworn body repaired, part by part, and had just gotten new knees when I last texted him holiday greetings in January 2018. He replied happily that he was renewed enough to live into his 80s. Only when I got the fall copy of "The Shrine," our high school fund-raising rag, and opened it to a half-page picture of him, did I learn that he had died three weeks after our winter texts. Did he die alone? I have no idea. "Of natural causes," the newspaper obituary said. But there was no chance to say goodbye. Or thank you. Or, in the words of sports talk-radio, "I'm sorry you got trapped in the Suckverse."

The third person was my old friend Marc, from over 40 years ago when we were both participants in an NEH summer seminar at the University of California, in heaven-on-earth Berkeley. I immediately took to both him and his wife Sara, and aspired to hang out with them. They were urbane and savvy. Marc had a wry Jewish wit and an extraordinary bank of knowledge about esoterica from ancient rhetoric to lesser-known soul singers to Apple fonts and culinary delights. Sara had a librarian's meticulously detailed expertise plus an eye for the ridiculous and a droll, understated way of pronouncing on it. We bonded over Napa wines, used bookstores, and the delights of ethnic restaurants. And we remained friends. I visited them in Ann Arbor every winter holiday to share news of the weird. In the early years, we had gourmet home-cooked meals late in the evening, then drank into the wee hours. In later years, the food got tamer, the drinking more temperate, the bedtime hour earlier, but we remained friends. When Sara died in 2004 at the age of 59 and Marc was diagnosed with Parkinson's the same year, it was a terrible blow.

Marc gathered himself admirably to forge a new life. He bought a spacious apartment in Paris' Marais and acquired a new-old girlfriend who was equally wry, if less endearing. I visited them in Paris several times over the years, savoring the charms of leisurely life. After she too died a few years ago, Marc, with a residency permit, decided to live permanently in France because it was more affordable for those needing care homes and fulltime assistance. Because his condition had deteriorated so much, Marc had to strap his large body together to prevent its flailing when we walked down the street. And going two blocks was his upper limit. But we had good conversations and treasured the comfort of our long friendship.

A month ago, while cleaning out my desk, I found a postcard with Marc's name and Marais address scrolled on it. Suddenly I had an uncanny feeling that he was no longer alive. He had not responded to my last few emails, though I attributed that to advanced Parkinson's. When I researched obituaries online, as one does, it didn't take long to find him in the University of Chicago magazine. He had died in September 2019—several months ago. Because he had neither family nor children, no one had sent out a notice. Sadly, he too may have died alone.

Where does grief go, when there are no rituals to voice and mourn it? I feel it, hanging like a dead weight, black and still, over my head. Recently I heard a *This American Life* segment (#597), "One Last Thing before I Go," on how grief is being expressed for those who died in the tsunami and earthquake that hit Japan with violent waves in 2011.[10] It killed over 19,000 people, and thousands more went missing. In one town, Otsuchi, people found a way to connect to them. A man, Itaru, mourning a lost cousin, had placed an old-fashioned white telephone booth, with a rotary phone that no longer worked, in his garden on a hill overlooking the Pacific. He named it "the wind telephone." It is used regularly by people who step inside it to "call" their departed relatives and carry on conversations about their feelings—of grief, anger, guilt—with the beloved family member. (Their calls were videotaped for a documentary commemorating the fifth anniversary of the tsunami.) Some weep, some rant. Some confide old secrets. Some calls are ordinary updates on the progress of life for the living. People wish their loved ones alive—somewhere—or voice their sadness about not having been able to save them. They reassure the dead that the living are doing okay, so that the dead will not worry and be stuck in no-man's land. This sharing seems to bring comfort, although the telephone can't really connect them.

Now, thousands from all over Japan come to use the phone. In Buddhism, the border between the living and the dead is said to be thinner than in the west. Connection happens.

At this time, perhaps the biggest loss is the difficulty of finding a way to connect again with those who have left. And then, how do we connect to ourselves?

Early May 2020: Becoming Feral

Eight weeks into Coronaville, the things that first seemed bizarre—wearing a mask to go grocery shopping, seeing almost no one, renouncing movies and restaurants for TV and dinners at home—are becoming, if not normal, The Way It Is. Where I once defined my days around going to the gym for aqua aerobics or dance exercise and savoring the weekly bridge meet-up, the occasional university lecture, the movies, and cocktails on Saturday night, my ambition now is to carve out the day to include a walk of at least a half hour at a reasonably brisk pace. Grocery-shopping twice a week—Wednesday and Friday or Saturday—is the adventurous highlight. All those things are hangovers from The Before Time.

And we are in Now. It was a novelty at first to watch TV shows where men in jackets or shirtsleeves stood up at the end to reveal their boxer shorts. (There is no analogue to this for women.) And the glimpses of their kitchens and home offices that seemed stolen are now part of a show's expected furniture. It would seem strange not to have that odd, awkward intimacy. On my end, I congratulate myself on still making an effort. But my rituals are few: a daily shower and straightening the comforter on my bed. I get out of my robe and pajamas once a day, but often at a latish hour. I wear sweats in nice color combinations—rose pink with violet, red and navy, gray and black—but have worn nothing else for the duration. Once a week I change them, whether they need it or not. Bra? Nah. Stretchy tube-tops do well enough, and socks must be changed—every second day. The slacker life.

I've never liked washing my hair but do it religiously once a week. Can't say I comb it but I run a hand through it daily, and wish it were long enough to pull into a ponytail. I was growing my dirty-blonde color out and letting silver invade it like a patch of weeds, but now it's a runaway train, curling in wild abandon. Think Steven Pinker on a bad day or, more likely, Albert Einstein. I've discovered the great American secret—if you put on a baseball cap when going out, nobody knows about your hair (which explains why at least half my students in the past decade came to class with caps on their heads).

I was on a downward spiral with dressing anyway—since I retired almost six years ago, I segued to black LuluLemon pants with a black T-shirt, and tossed on some kind of jacket. You can go anywhere in that, just alter the layers and lengths for winter or summer. But now those clothes would be my "dress" outfit—too close-fitting, asking for too much maintenance against cat hair. On a recent "Fresh Air with Terry Gross" radio show, fashion guru Tim Gunn admitted that he now lives in a white T-shirt, pajama bottoms, and a navy bathrobe and that putting on "street clothes" felt like wearing a wetsuit. Meanwhile 95% of the clothes in my closet hang abandoned. Will it ever be possible to wear them again? It will feel like strapping on a corset. (And yes, I probably have bulges in a few places that used to be lean—in these days, cookies are essential.)

Part of what's great about sweats is that they truly go everywhere, always appropriate for a walk in the woods, acceptable in the grocery store where all eyes are fixed on which mask one is wearing—or not. I fantasize about writing on mine, "I'm wearing this to protect you. Please return the favor." But it's Ohio and there's no telling if I'd be punched. And make-up? Lipstick seems superfluous—just soils the mask. Eyeliner has been de rigueur; but when people are at least six feet away, is it even visible? Perfume? If I started sniffling from my fragrance, or someone else's, it would seem like a symptom. Its main use now is to check if we can still smell scents.

Women's fashion magazines used to celebrate "the fresh face," which meant denuded of make-up, as if you'd just wandered out of the woods. But when you've really just wandered out, the effect is altogether different. Truly windblown and scruffy at the edges, perhaps a bit ripe.

Closer to the animal world. Going feral.

How bad could that be? Animals are said to be joyously reclaiming the streets. I live in a city so I see mostly children (definitely looking feral as they wade in creeks and yell with abandon) and small creatures like bunnies and squirrels. The imagination of living among animals, lost to us for so long, is no longer just a dream.

One of my favorite parts of a little wood I frequent near home is the walk along Slyh Run, where someone has cunningly constructed three forts from tree boughs and sticks. They are built like tepees, with vertical stakes crossing at the top and horizontal ones woven around them to define the space of rooms. One is large enough that I can stand up in it. At first, I thought they were built as shelters by homeless people, but nothing changes in them from day to day. I've stepped inside and thought about what it would be like to live in the woods, sleep on the dirt, and watch the stars through the pointed roof, rising with the sun and building a little fire in the stone- ringed pit to heat water. We're not deep enough in the country, of course—but it does seem like one more step toward returning to some primal union with the natural world.

But that easy romance is deceptive. I lived that way once, for the better part of three years—and it was gritty, itchy, and lonely. Simple things—a hot shower, a reading lamp, putting on shoes without shaking them for spiders or scorpions—became yearned-for moments. And we did become more than a bit feral. Going into town—a dusty two-bit Oklahoma town in Pushmataha County without even a movie theater or library, but more than one liquor store—while standing in a check-out line, we would idly scratch the fierce chigger bites on our stomachs that lasted over a month. We become the stereotype of hicks. But I had learned how to live in the woods. Sitting in the Cherokee Jeep with the dog on my lap for long drives on dirt paths to our camp, I would pass time by pulling ticks from her coat that had filled up with enough blood to be lifted easily. Out the window they went, while she whimpered. When I had to, I killed a copperhead with a shovel. And tarantulas. When armadillos snorted and prodded the sides of our tent in the middle of the night, I felt neither revulsion nor fear. Only my partner's scratching in his sleep could wake me up—to poke him to stop.

I thought that not many traces of that early-80s time remained in my routine, but some have returned now. The compost pile, the stash of toilet paper, water, and canned food. Recently I made what is called a bug-out bag for when you have to leave home at once—because of a tornado, an anthrax attack, a bomb. It is staunchly unglamorous and practical, full of things like goggles, bandages, a multitask knife, a space blanket. I debate whether to get a weapon, perhaps a stun gun. But that seems like crossing a line—from feral to brutal.

20 May 2020: Back to the World

Generally, I don't think much about The Before Time because I'm not missing it. The pleasures of being truly and irretrievably home are exquisite, if subtle. On my daily walk, there are few cars on the road, and I pass increasing numbers of neighbors walking. So much feels like long ago—perhaps my youth in the Fifties. Other than changes in clothing styles, it is hard to tell. Life is at a slower, more leisurely pace, as we drink in colors and smells, enjoying the sheer pleasure of movement. Yet there is also computer enhancement to monitor news and deal with the ongoing overload of academic email. Some days I calibrate all the things that have gotten broken, outmoded, or gone missing in my house—a new seeing. And nearly every evening, there is a real phone call with a friend or relative. It's like the 1980s, when phone chats were a delicious ritual, before the internet commandeered our lives.

This is stripped-down living, of course. No movies, no theatre, no dancing. No dinner parties, no sitting in cozy bars having a drink. No estate sales or library visits. No gym workouts or dreamy massages. No art or music or . . . so much more. Worst of all, no fun, cuddly visits with the grandchildren. But I live a privileged life, unlike so many, and I am healthy, reasonably well off, and like living as an introvert. Yet I wonder—will we all go crazy after another month? Or just stay a bit furry, ding-y, and cabin-fevered?

Still, I realized today that many stores are open. So, I ventured out. I found myself becoming enraged at shoppers who don't wear masks—as if they're playing Russian roulette with not only their own but also others' lives. I smile at the masked, then realize they can't see the smile behind my own mask. Later, I will learn to look to their eyes and body language for signals of solidarity, or at least compliance. But those little gestures came gradually, as we learned the alternative codes of living in a world ravaged by disease. Today, entering with my mask firmly on, I wonder if it is okay to touch things? Just browsing the racks makes me feel slightly guilty—isn't this non-essential? And what IS essential? I could wear sweatpants for the rest of my life, as I have for the last two months, and would be acceptably and decently covered.

After he retired in the Seventies, my father, who had always worn a suit and tie with a dapper hat on his bald head, shifted to jogging suits, what were then called "leisure suits"—two of them, one navy, the other emerald-green. Except for the rare times when he left the house, he never wore anything else. It seemed strange to me then, but now it makes sense. The jogging suits were like a skin. Enough.

7 July 2020: News of the Weird

Perhaps the strangest thing about these times is that they are now only intermittently weird. How easily we accommodate to change! There are moments when I catch myself in the grocery store staring at shelves that are still bare of some things. Now, it's rice cakes, my preferred breakfast food, with good Irish butter, and there are no LED light bulbs, but toilet paper and paper towels are suddenly abundant. Much, in the intense summer heat and lush growth, seems "normal." Nature is in full frolic, the birds singing madly and much louder than in previous years. Deer are crowding the fringes of the city. The cats lounge outside, basking in the sun.

The other night I watched a penumbral moon that, by midnight, was a diffuse orange ball of compelling light. The small clouds that sailed across it like black darts. Driven by its lunatic force I felt like an animal ready to prowl on the ground, with the cats. Driving home on the freeway from a friend's, I couldn't get my car lights to work—inexplicably it was brighter when they were off, yet still not very bright. I wasn't enough an animal to see by the light of the moon, even a full one. Driving with only moonlight, I felt reckless. Turning at my exit I went off the road to allow the car pressing me from behind to pass me—and into the gravel, almost landing in a ditch.

I made it home, navigating near-empty streets, wondering if my eyes had gone dim. Or had the car lights somehow reversed themselves, so that "on" was "off" and vice versa? That would be an apt metaphor for these times. The next morning, though it was a Sunday, when I contacted her, my ophthalmologist advised me to see a retinal specialist, given that I am almost legally blind in my left eye (which matters not at all when gazing at the moon). Gradually it occurred to me that the fault could be in our stars, as Cassius said to Brutus. What if it was the lights, not I, that had gone out? But if I threw money at it, all would be good again.

It's a case in point. Although little oddities are not the focus of the days as long as I stay home—in my humble castle with its endless imperial demands to fix, throw out, upgrade—they stud its careless moments. The day-to-day goes along, with the weird burrowed in it. It's like the movie *Groundhog Day*—each day runs its course of waking rituals, meals, chores, work, little pleasures—going to the grocery store, the resale, seeing each grandkid once a week. I do not scorn these pleasures; they are familiar and comforting. But the day's prospects are always the same. There is no possibility that a crack will open to let something new and surprisingly wonderful emerge. (This is a challenge to the universe—prove me wrong!) But the weird also has a sense of humor that calls to us. We live like bugs in the garden retreading familiar routes—till smashed, sprayed with toxin, killed by cold. Ah, that's not so funny! More Gregor Samsa-like.

And if COVID has been good for anything, it's reviving Kafka's sense of the absurd and unpredictable entwined with daily life, usually leading to a dire end. (*The Trial*'s [1925] last words, when Josef K. is executed, are: "Like a dog."[11]) And Kierkegaard, with his sense of existential risk in *Fear and Trembling* (1843). They were writers I devoured as an undergraduate in the sixties and have rarely read since. If routine allows, I'll read more of Knausgaard's endless Nordic self-reflections. It's a good time for the perplexes of K's.

Fall 2020: Thinking Covidiously

These five months have been a time of reckoning with the material accumulation of decades. Surely mine, as a collector intrigued by many things—books, postcards, fabrics, vintage pitchers and jugs, clothes, shoes, African art, tin boxes and signs, movies on DVD, and on and on—is substantial and of great significance to me, if no one else. (A friend visiting my house for the first time said she felt like she was in a museum—I didn't ask what kind.) But the agglomeration was beginning to feel stifling and, I, like so many other Marie Kondo'ed self-critics, felt, in my bones of Baroque Catholic excess, that Puritan strain rising up to purge and feel virtuous. And we are numerous—every time I go to the Goodwill with another load, people are emptying trunks full of household goods. If the retail market collapses in the coming year, we will all be able to resupply in thrift stores.

It is easy to begin cleaning out some category of house-junk and end up playing with it like children playing house. But a friend and I have discovered a way to tackle the mounds of unmentionables without getting lost or discouraged. We come to each other's house on alternate Friday afternoons. These are not casual purge-visits, but a formal, even ritualized, process of identifying and completing one task per week. It's social, satisfying, almost virtuous. We are careful but not masked. The pleasure of hours of conversation with a friend! In its own small way, our ritual feels like a response to a broader sense of disorder—a counter to the chaos, isolation, and uncertainty that have come to define collective experiences of plague.

There is a Western genealogy of plague literature from Thucydides through Boccaccio's *Decameron* to Daniel Defoe's *Journal of the Plague Year* (1722) and Camus's *The Plague*. Plague also intrudes in novels from Chinua Achebe's *Things Fall Apart* (1958) to Chimamanda Ngozi Adichie's *Half of a Yellow Sun* (2006). In agrarian African societies, raging communicable diseases can be as common as seasonal cycles. Insect plagues—the "plague of locusts"—barely merit mention. And what of Ebola, that ravaging, flesh-eating disease that truly destroys its victims? Other than general alarm when an American nurse brought it into the country, it was a blip on American radar. Malaria, which continues to afflict much of Africa, southeast Asia, and parts of Central America, hasn't been designated a plague because it recurs annually with predictable regularity. And yet, as recently as three decades ago, 28.2% of children under five in West Africa died from it.[12]

The modern West used to distinguish itself from these "plague-ridden" parts of the developing world. But the politics of COVID troubles this binary. On the right are the public deniers who subscribe to the Trump-endorsed social media line that the pandemic will disappear the day after the election is held. A small group of them, in Army fatigues and carrying firearms, some were wearing masks, many were not, stormed the State House in Lansing, Michigan,[13] and the capitals of several other states to protest public shutdown rules and curfews as infringement on their right of free assembly. It became clear that such public protests were only an opening salvo to bolder plans, such as kidnapping Michigan Governor Gretchen Whitmer, and casting her adrift on a boat in the middle of a lake.[14] Notably, this plan—hatched in Ohio—was not an isolated incident, but part of a broader, coordinated network of conspirators across the Rustbelt, underscoring how deeply embedded such extremism remains in the region.

But it isn't only in America that these tensions have surfaced. What of the hordes of protesters who gather in cities—London, Berlin, Paris—to protest governmental rules restricting public gatherings as the pandemic escalates to new, virulent heights this November? Are they NIMBYs who support the welfare of all except when it gets in their way? Suddenly they seem more like the American wild west with its mantra, "Don't fence me in."

Beyond these protests and politics, we might ask: What are the aesthetics of COVID beyond decorated masks and good cartoons? It seems too soon to know what will emerge, except on the everyday front. Locally, and no doubt internationally, there's an explosion of silver hair on women who used to be blonde, red, or brunette. Interestingly it doesn't just look like "truth"—it looks good! And then there's what passes for style. I don't see women in heels, tight jeans, and shapely jackets these days—it's sweat pants, braless tops, and sneakers since March. I mean really—if you're wearing a mask and glasses, what difference does it make? And something has to give for that extra five pounds.

What is a pandemic good for? It is easy and customary to bemoan losses. In lives and quality of life, they are indeed grievous and massive, scandalously massive, in the United States. Yet the quarantining around this epidemic has brought things into personal life that we are discovering we have missed.

A Long, Strange Trip: Halloween 2020

When the babysitter of one of my grandchildren contracted the virus, I insisted on getting tested, despite my doctor's assurance that I didn't need to. I drove to the giant Ohio Fairgrounds building that has been turned into a drive-through testing spot, a cross between a car wash and a drive-in movie. Through my car window I was given the test—a quick, painless swab just inside the nose. Then, I drove off, assuming my result the next day would be a non-event. But to my shock, the MyChart communiqué read, "You have tested positive for Covid." On the list of status rankings, mine was "abnormal." It seemed to be the lowest ranking; there were also heavy and very heavy categories. But the message was clear: "Quarantine in isolation for 10 days."

I was stunned. The test had to be wrong! Perhaps I had a few symptoms—a bit of sore throat and achiness—irritations that were vague and not debilitating. But, no, my doctor said that I'd had the PCR test, currently the most precise.

In fact, there are few guidelines on how to isolate. Veterinarians caution against cuddling pets because the virus can be passed to other mammals, especially cats. So much for emotional-support animals. I had stocked up on food, drink, and, yes, toilet paper, with a sense of impending unease in the wake of the election. But there was no time to be bored. Television had endlessly entertaining Scandi-krimis, and in between was putt-putt work to clean up the gardens for winter. My inner nun rejoiced as I finished little projects and slept more than usual. There were strangely few symptoms: my throat hurt and I had an upper backache that I ascribed to having wrenched my right shoulder. I later discovered that such aches—described by afflicted actor Hugh Grant as a feeling as though an enormous man was sitting on his chest—are typical. But I had no cough or runny nose; I could smell and taste as acutely as ever. And, while a little tired and momentarily dizzy at times, I was neither short of breath nor feverish. It was time in isolation, but it was not a Big Deal.

When I called my brother, a retired cardiologist living up on Lake Ontario, to report my Covid diagnosis, his response was, "That's good news!" He explained that I would now have a degree of immunity as we enter the impending dark days of this winter. "The only problem is," he added, "you'll be a leper."

Indeed. I've experienced what feels like "victim-shaming" from a few people. And I've learned to say nothing of the illness in casual conversation; if asked how I am, I'm "fine." We're all masked and distanced. Only I know that, in a given group, I'm the safest one to be near because I am, for a few months, immune. (My doctor wrote that I am "no longer infectious and only shedding dead virus, and most likely have developed antibodies to COVID-19.") I carry with me a letter from the Office of Infectious Disease Investigation of the local Department of Health:

> This letter is to inform you that as of 11/17/2020 you have been released from home isolation.
>
> You are under no travel restrictions and you can return to your normal work or school activities. You may share this letter with your employer as a confirmation that you are no longer considered to be contagious.

The letter was signed "Elexia," which one witty friend speculated was an Artificial Intelligence cousin of Amazon's Alexa. As to "contact tracing," it seems well intended but ineffectual. Three days after my diagnosis, the Department of Health left a phone message; when I returned it, no one answered. The next day I got a call from "Lexi" asking me if I would like them to contact my family. "No," I replied, "I've done that." End of conversation.

So, the leper returns to society—at least until the next time that, perish the thought, I contract the virus. (Yes, it's possible, and eventually would happen.) A few traces of the experience remain. If I overdo and start to tire, it hits like a bomb. And that peculiar COVID dizziness still sneaks up once in a while, making me sit down fast. It feels like I've been displaced from my body, jangling the border of flesh and air. Although I was never exactly sick, now I'm not exactly well. There's a weird sensitivity in not just my throat and eyes but, *pace* Leonard Cohen, the places where I used to play. The recovery is less a bounce-back than a crawl-back. But, Dr. G reassures me, that's what viruses do. Give it a month or two. (*Or two?*)

Most days I'm stronger and feeling the comfort of short-term immunity. In retrospect, an undercurrent of dread colored my days over the past months. There are good reasons for it—COVID can be severe and life-destroying. Even in the best of situations, such as mine, it hangs around long after the contagion period, a reminder of how fragile mortality is. We begin to learn how life was changed in past plague times.

What does all this mean in the larger scope of things? Unquestionably, it breeds compassion for others who are afflicted with COVID, and a sense of horror at how grave the illness can be. Such phrases as "dying alone" take on concrete and hallucinatory meaning. My admiration grows for "essential workers," doctors and nurses, and also teachers, grocery clerks, garbage collectors, taxi and bus drivers, airline workers, janitors. What erupted in my body as an unexpected and annoying, but ultimately minor, surprise is a sword hanging over their heads day by day—and felling too many. In a small way, I am starting to understand what COVID survivors mean when they say, "I want my life back."

April 2020: Back to the Beginning

In April 2020, at the start of the pandemic, I wrote a list for an online project of a pandemic archive called *Coronavirus Lost and Found.*[15] Little did I know how persistent and true those initial impressions would become. My "quaranzine" becomes truer with each passing month:

Lost: My great recreation center, where I alternated aqua aerobics classes in a warm-water pool with fitness-dance classes till the sweat began to break.

Found: My neighborhood, where I've lived for over 12 years and am only now discovering on walks. There is a little wood in one direction, a tiny creek-walk in the opposite. In between, lots of burby houses, humble on my side of the dividing road, more upscale-landscaped on the other side. Now, in mid-Ohio early spring, the profusion of wildflowers, trees in bud and bloom, changes almost daily, moving from daffodils to hyacinths to tulips to lilacs. The wild beauty of spring is almost too much to bear.

Lost: My wonderful funded trip to Europe, with days of research in Amsterdam and Berlin, a workshop and an international autobiography conference in Finland, and, as a reward for all that virtue, a trip to St. Petersburg, with a stay in a brilliant hotel during the White Nights of June.

Found: Tove Jansson's "Moomin" comics and stories, which I read in preparation for

Finland. She was the extraordinary, imaginative creator of the alternative Moomin world of blobby folk-animal-creatures living in a communal hodgepodge who annually emerged from nine months of winter to have mind-bending adventures in Moominland. Reading these books is close to perfect happiness. And the Petersburg hotel refunded my exorbitant deposit when I mentioned I was a senior—they decided in my favor because of my "venerable age," referring to me as a "babushka." I prefer "venerable."

Lost: My family, including local grandkids who are seven and three, the light of my life, for the indefinite future. FaceTime and waving through their picture window just aren't enough.

Found: Phone conversations and exchanges with friends around the world and from decades past who are warm and caring. The family we make . . .

Lost: Artists, intellectuals, ordinary people. Luckily as yet none from my big Irish family, still with 12 cousins—but some are so fragile.

Found: The pleasure of singing along to every word of every song on John Prine's *Diamonds in the Rough*—while mourning his COVID-related death.

Lost: My dirty-blonde-colored bob.

Found: My silver curls.

Lost: The ease of living in a reasonably predictable world.

Found: Deep sadness that sometimes slams into my head like a brick.

Notes

1 Alison Bechdel, quoted in Ted Loos, "What Has Lockdown Meant for L.G.B.T.Q. Artists and Writers?" *The New York Times*, June 16, 2020, https://www.nytimes.com/2020/06/16/arts/gay- lgbt-artists-coronavirus-theater-dance.html.
2 Bechdel, qtd. in Loos, "What Has Lockdown Meant."
3 Lynda Barry, "Documenting All the Small Things That Are Easily Lost," *New York Times*, May 1, 2020.
4 Leslie Jamison, "When the World Went Away, We Made a New One," *New York Times*, May 19, 2020.
5 Jon Pareless, "John Prine, Who Chronicled the Human Condition in Song, Dies at 73," *New York Times*, April 7, 2020, https://www.nytimes.com/2020/04/07/arts/music/john-prine-dead- coronavirus.html.
6 Jamison, "When the World Went Away."
7 Deborah Eisenberg, "Awful but Joyful," *The New York Review*, March 25, 2021.
8 Sidonie Smith and Julia Watson, "Autobiographical Reckonings in America's Restless Twenty-First Century," in *The Divided States: Unraveling National Identities in the Twenty-First Century*, ed. Laura J. Beard and Ricia Anne Chansky (Madison: University Wisconsin Press, 2023), 297.

9 Leanne Italie and Emily Leshner, "Death Cafés Help Ease Grief, Loss," *Chicago Sun-Times*, July 1, 2020.
10 Ira Glass, host, "One Last Thing Before I Go," *This American Life*, episode 597, September 23, 2016. WBEZ Chicago, https://www.thisamericanlife.org/597/one-last-thing-before-i-go-2016.
11 Franz Kafka, *The Trial*, trans. David Wyllie (Project Gutenberg, 2005), n.p.
12 Robert W. Snow and Judy A. Omumbo, "Malaria," in *Disease and Mortality in Sub-Saharan Africa*, ed. Dean Jamison et al. (Nih.gov, The International Bank for Reconstruction and Development, The World Bank, 2025), https://www.ncbi.nlm.nih.gov/books/NBK2286/#A1238.
13 Craig Mauger, "Protesters, Some Armed, Enter Michigan Capitol in Rally Against COVID-19 Limits," *The Detroit News*, April 30, 2020.
14 Nicholas Bogel Burroughs, Shaila Dewan, and Kathleen Gray, "F.B.I. Says Michigan Anti-Government Group Plotted to Kidnap Gov. Gretchen Whitmer," *The New York Times*, October 8, 2020.
15 Julia Watson, "Something Found for Each Thing Lost," *Coronavirus Lost and Found*, April 2020, https://pandemicarchive.com/something-found-for-each-thing-lost/.

Bibliography

Barry, Lynda. "Documenting All the Small Things That Are Easily Lost." *The New York Times*, May 1, 2020. https://www.nytimes.com/2020/05/01/arts/lynda-barry-diary-project.html.

Bechdel, Alison. Quoted in "What Has Lockdown Meant for L.G.B.T.Q. Artists and Writers?" Ted Loos, *The New York Times*, June 16, 2020. https://www.nytimes.com/2020/06/16/arts/gay-lgbt-artists-coronavirus-theater-dance.html.

Ditlevsen, Tove. *The Copenhagen Trilogy: Childhood-Youth-Dependency (1959–61)*. Translated by Michael Favala Goldman. New York: Farrar, Straus and Giroux, 2021.

Eisenberg, Deborah. "Awful but Joyful." *The New York Review*, March 25, 2021. https://www.nybooks.com/articles/2021/03/25/tove-ditlevsen-awful-but-joyful/?lp_txn_id=1614388.

Italie, Leanne, and Emily Leshner. "Death Cafés Help Ease Grief, Loss." *Chicago Sun-Times*, July 1, 2020. https://chicago.suntimes.com/2020/7/1/21310822/death-cafes-help-ease-grief- coronavirus.

Jamison, Leslie. "When the World Went Away, We Made a New One." *The New York Times*, May 19, 2020. https://www.nytimes.com/interactive/2020/05/19/magazine/covid-quarantine- recovery.html.

Smith, Sidonie, and Julia Watson. "Autobiographical Reckonings in America's Restless Twenty-First Century." In *The Divided States: Unraveling National Identities in the Twenty-First Century*, edited by Laura J. Beard and Ricia Anne Chansky, 296–324. Madison: University of Wisconsin Press, 2023.

Snow, Robert W., and Judy A Omumbo. "Malaria." In *Disease and Mortality in Sub-Saharan Africa*, edited by Dean Jamison et al. Nih.gov, The International Bank for Reconstruction and Development, The World Bank, 2025. www.ncbi.nlm.nih.gov/books/NBK2286/#A1238.

Watson, Julia. "Something Found for Each Thing Lost." *Coronavirus Lost and Found*, April 2020. https://pandemicarchive.com/something-found-for-each-thing-lost/.

2

"I IMAGINE THE CIRCUMSTANCES OF MY DEATH"

Life Writing as Radical Absence in Kate Baer's COVID-19-Era Poetry

Irene Gammel and Jason Wang

"I imagine the circumstances of my death," writes Kate Baer in her poem "At the Covid Testing Clinic," distilling the existential precarity of pandemic life into a single, haunting line.[1] The COVID-19 pandemic upended daily life and forced writers to grapple with trauma. From Kitty O'Meara's ode to stillness "And the People Stayed Home" ("And they listened, and read books, and rested,/. . ./and learned new ways of being"),[2] to Richard Hendrick's mediative "Lockdown" ("They say that in the streets of Assisi/People are singing to each other"),[3] pandemic poetry became a cultural archive of both resilience and despair. During a time when many poets suffered from writer's block,[4] this surge of verse was more than documentation: it redefined poetry's role as both literary form and social practice, collapsing boundaries between private anguish and public discourse.

Within this context, Kate Baer's pandemic-era poetry collections—*What Kind of Woman* (2020), *I Hope This Finds You Well* (2021), and *And Yet* (2022)—stand out for their radical interrogation of silences and erasure. By redacting hostile messages, political rhetoric, and digital noise, Baer transforms erasure into a feminist poetics of resistance, reclaiming agency amid the dual crises of COVID-19 and patriarchal governance. This chapter argues that Baer's work reimagines erasure as a mode of life writing—one that exposes systemic silences while crafting a fragmented, palimpsestic selfhood. Drawing on digital marginalia in relation to life writing, her poetry performs a dual critique: it illuminates the erasures enacted by pandemic precarity and misogynistic discourse, while asserting autonomy through strategic deletions. Her texts—often born from social media exchanges—reframe digital detritus as lyrical testimony, blurring the lines between poet, speaker, and reader. In doing so, Baer challenges traditional life writing's linearity, offering instead a discontinuous subjectivity shaped by absence as much as by presence. Drawing on feminist archival and life writing theories, we focus on Baer's

DOI: 10.4324/9781003735595-4

contribution to pandemic literature, positioning erasure poetry as a critical tool for navigating the tension between hypervisibility and silencing in the digital age. Baer's subtractive aesthetics forge a counter-historiography, in which what is withheld speaks as powerfully as what remains.

Baer's work is part of a larger poetic response to the crisis, as poetry surged to prominence during the COVID-19 pandemic and was frequently preserved in later-published print anthologies. *Singing in the Dark: A Global Anthology of Poetry under Lockdown* (2020), edited by K. Satchidanandan and Nisha Chawla, gathers over a hundred poets from more than 20 countries, offering a snapshot of the pandemic's early phase and its transformative impact on everyday life. *Get Lost Dirty COVID-19!* (2020) presents an Australian mother-daughter collaboration between academic Zuivere Mamgain and eighth-grader Madalsa Mamgain. In one poem, Madalsa mourns the loss of her childhood—"a piece of my child heart is dying every day"—while her mother reflects on her own mortality as friends die, weaving generational perspectives into a shared narrative of grief and resilience.[5]

Literary scholars have been quick to recognize poetry as a cultural hallmark of the pandemic. As Lauren Bravo observes: "It's being retweeted at pace, shared by distant friends on Facebook and slipped into our pockets via WhatsApp groups."[6] Drawing on reader response data, linguist Marcello Giovanelli argues that COVID-19 poetry acts as both a personal and social record of the pandemic's emotional and psychological toll. Unlike fiction, which may offer escapism, such poetry helps process grief, articulate anxiety, and provide solace. Giovanelli likens its cultural role to other forms of non-fictional crisis writing, underscoring poetry's power for emotional and communal expression. As COVID-19 poetry gained visibility as a socially embedded form, public humanities scholar Jeroen Dera notes a key shift.[7] He argues that the traditional divide between autonomous and heteronomous poetry—as theorized by scholars like Gisèle Sapiro and Pierre Bourdieu—is destabilized in moments of crisis creating tension. While some, like Belgian poet Delphine Lecompte, dismiss pandemic poetry as aesthetically weak, such critiques overlook how even formally unrefined poems, as Rita Felski observes, provoke strong affective and social responses. For Dera, readers engage COVID-19 poetry as both artistic form and personal experience—a hybrid mode enabling personal reflection and communal meaning-making, bridging the public and private. The pandemic, he argues, redefined poetry's cultural role, revealing its power to connect emotional expression with public discourse.

More recent work explores how COVID-19 poetry also serves as a form of emotional self-care, especially when aligned with life writing practices that confront the emotional and psychic costs of the pandemic. Communication scholar Daneshewar Sharma, for example, draws on her own poetic practice as a form of bibliotherapy and autotherapy to discuss how poetry helped her cope with fear and uncertainty during the pandemic.[8] Likewise, Judith Blundell and Simon Poole emphasize the mental health benefits of reading and writing poetry to foster "positive wellbeing,"[9] while psychologist Ahron Friedberg mobilizes COVID-19 poetry as a part of his therapeutic work with patients.[10]

In this broader landscape, we contend that Philadelphia poet Kate Baer redefines poetic erasure as a form of life writing that confronts the intertwined crises of the COVID-19 pandemic and Trump-era politics, reframing selfhood through subtractive resistance. By redacting hostile Instagram messages, presidential speeches, pandemic correspondence, and online harassment, Baer transforms toxic discourse into lyric testimonies of motherhood, digital labor, and collective grief. Positioned at the intersection of feminist life writing and critical poetry studies, this analysis draws on Andie Silva's concept of "digital marginalia" and Kate Eichhorn's archival poetics to theorize erasure as both a technology of self-representation and a political act. With this framework in place, we turn to a close reading of Baer's pandemic poetry, demonstrating how life writing during COVID-19 articulates resistance through an aesthetic of radical absence.

"2020"

Signaling autobiographical immersion in a specific historical moment of crisis, the one-word title of Baer's free verse poem "2020" sets the stage, speaking not just through what is said but what is absent. Even though COVID-19 is not mentioned, the poem evokes its world, beginning with a mundane object—coffee—and its fluctuating price, inviting empathic readings by those undergoing similar experiences.

> we complain about the price of coffee
> as if it isn't becoming extinct
> along with the rest of us
> would it be so wrong if we cut off every billionaire at the knees would it be so wrong if
> I touched my face to yours two men run for office
> it doesn't matter who they've ruined
> this is the year I unfriend anyone who uses a beauty filter
> who fetishizes youth into social currency
> . . .
> I don't know
> how we manage our ordinary lives
> when we're this close to the death in dying
> go ahead and tell me otherwise
> go ahead and tell me something good[11]

The poem responds to the twin upheavals of 2020—the pandemic and the US election—braiding health and political crises. With bluntness, the speaker voices anger at economic inequality ("cut off every billionaire at the knees") and political apathy ("two men run for office/it doesn't matter who they've ruined").[12]

The speaker's frustration, grief, and weariness capture the emotional toll of COVID-19, especially in the line "would it be so wrong if/I touched my face to yours," evoking the loss of physical contact under the physical distancing rules. This deprivation underscores the poem's focus on emotional and social fallout, rather than on the medical or scientific narratives that dominated public conversations.

The poem "2020" reflects on the apocalyptic atmosphere of the year, where global health crises, political instability, and climate anxiety converged. The lines "we complain about the price of coffee/as if it isn't becoming extinct/along with the rest of us" illustrate how small daily grievances persisted even as society faced existential threats. By thematizing the COVID-19 experience without naming it, Baer plays with presence and absence, grappling with the aesthetic form, which is evident in her use of pronouns that help Baer negotiate individual and collective identity: the self-representational "I" and the politically positioned "we" emphasize issues of personal vulnerability, isolation, and care. The poem opens with the collective "we complain," framing the speaker's concerns as communal in tumultuous times. This collective invocation precedes and contextualizes the six subsequent uses of "I" and "me," suggesting tension between personal and collective experiences. This movement between "I" and "we" is poignant in a poem concerned with communicable illness and national stakes (via both the election and the pandemic).

This tension continues in "this is the year I unfriend/anyone who uses a beauty filter," where highly personal choices and reactions contribute to the poem's deeply autobiographical tone of irritation and resistance. The poem works as a documentary archive—a site of politicized assembly and disassembly, similar to the archive described by feminist archival scholar Kate Eichhorn: a space where what is lost, suppressed, or erased becomes central.[13] The speaker's decision to "unfriend" performs a pointed act of digital curation and refusal, echoing Eichhorn's notion of fragmentation as a political practice of contemporary documentation, as a strategy to resist dominant systems. Erasure, absence, and fragmentation thus serve as both aesthetic and political strategies, especially in feminist and activist contexts. These gestures of deletion and resistance to beautified online identities critique visibility, capitalism, and digital mediation through personal revolt.

Through silence—by keeping the crisis unspoken—Baer's aesthetic distancing strategies operate through ostensible gaps approximating those of other poets seeking to communicate trauma or taboo (like the stark, cavernous gaps found in Canadian childhood sexual abuse survivor poems discussed by literary scholar Natalie Cooke[14]). In the end, Bear's lines "I don't know/how we manage our ordinary lives/when we're this close to the death in dying" dramatically reframe daily life in relation to death, with uncertainty—"I don't know"—figuring as a hallmark of life writing, the "I" affirming existence as highly precarious, configured by what is not known, like the uncertainty of illness and death. This poem's substraction strategy—from its minimalist title to its ostensible omission of all punctuation—makes the experiences jumble together, reflecting the autobiographical messiness of real-life. Moreover, the removal of all upper-case letters at the beginning of sentences suggests unprocessed immediacy: urgent, vulnerable, and raw stream-of-consciousness spilling out during crisis. The final lines, "go ahead and tell me otherwise/go ahead and tell me something good," shift to a "you" is a double-edged challenge: on one hand, opening the door for comfort but, on the other, the taunting tone making it clear that any answer might be met with mistrust. This frustration invites readers to sit with the speaker's weariness and doubt, and to consider how collective experiences of uncertainty and isolation shape the way we listen, respond, and care. This distancing aesthetic is further highlighted in her poem "Unsettling," which turns to one of the pandemic's most visible and contested symbols: the face mask—a symbol of in/visibility.

"Unsettling"

Masked teller.
Masked shopper.
Masked baby.
Masked butcher.
Masked runner.
Masked neighbor.
Masked lover.
Masked wife.[15]

Contrasting with the previous poem's use of "I" and "we," "Unsettled" strips the poem of all pronouns and verbs, creating a bare list presented as an octave. The eight-times repeated "Masked" anaphora amplifies the mask as the most dominant visual signifier of the pandemic. As the speaker lists encounters—"Masked teller./Masked shopper./Masked baby"—she captures the estrangement of COVID-19 social life in the absence of verbs in the poem's fragmented sentences, each line isolating each figure and heightening the sense of disconnection. The poem's minimalist structure emphasizes atomization: sentence fragments with only masked subjects, paralyzed and constrained, each isolated in its own line unit and end-stopped with a period, visually mimicking the familiar COVID-19 image line-ups of masked people—each separated by six feet—waiting in front of stores or in waiting rooms.

This flattening of identity mirrors the mask's paradoxical function: a barrier that simultaneously conceals (erasing expressions, muffling voices) and hyper-exposes (marking bodies as potential threats). "As a subject, the face mask gained new values and meanings in semantic, economic, political, fashion and cultural terms," observe Martina Topić, Marija Geiger Zeman, and Ivo Pilar in their study "Multiple Meanings of the Face Mask: Masking as the New Social Practice in the Context of Lockdown Creativity and Pandemic Chic."[16] Baer's repetition does more than underscore safety protocols; it formalizes the alienation of pandemic life, where human connection became a negotiation of risk. The poem's sparse, detached tone—a hallmark of her distancing aesthetic—reflects not just the physical act of masking but also the psychological residue of a society forced to equate proximity with danger. By framing the mask as both shield and shroud, Baer crystallizes the era's central tension: the collision of collective survival and the erosion of personhood.

As an octave, this short poem evokes the structure of the Petrarchan sonnet, in which the first eight lines pose a problem that the sestet traditionally resolves. But here, the sestet is missing, and the problem remains unresolved. The truncated form distills complex emotions into a compressed space, its abbreviated structure mirroring the disorientation of the pandemic and suggesting formal experimentation amid widespread disruption. A pattern of slant rhymes—the half rhymes of the "*er*" sounding at the end of tell*er*, shopp*er*, butch*er*, runn*er*, neighb*or*, and even lov*er*—creates a sense of strained predictability that is ostensibly resisted by two words: *baby* and *wife*. Their sonic non-compliance makes them stand out, marking them as sites of deeper emotional or social complexity, with the final phrase, "masked wife," signaling that the mask is both literal and symbolic, alluding to the masking performance expected of a wife at home. It mediates identity and obligation. Though the poet-speaker never says "I," her central stating of the roles of "masked lover" and "masked wife"—and the overlap with the poet's own roles as a wife and lover—suggest self-representational, embodied identities, with the mask rendering the body what life writing scholars Sidonie Smith and Julia Watson call "the site of autobiographical knowledge."[17] Just as the word "wife" stands out, so does the word "baby," with motherhood emerging as another axis of gendered identity under pressure—especially during the pandemic—as shown in the next poem.

"A Tired Mother in Pandemic Times"

With her experience raising four young children, Baer's poetry frequently addresses the realities of motherhood, often targeting what Spicher Kasdorf describes as "the insidious societal messages" surrounding its sentimentalization.[18] During the pandemic—when motherhood took on renewed urgency and women were burdened with double and triple roles in the domestic sphere—Baer released her second poetry collection, *I Hope This Finds You Well* (2021). Her focus on motherhood remained central, and her technique of poetic substraction sharpened as a form of resistance. As she explains in her prologue: "It wasn't until last year, when my first book was coming out and my inbox was flooded, that I started to examine some of these messages a little more closely."[19] On impulse, she took a screenshot of a particularly harsh message, redacted it with a pen, and reposted it as an erasure poem.[20] The result: the original message on the left side of the page, her erasure poem on the right, framed by her poetic title. By incorporating this public feedback loop[21]—feminist, misogynistic, even body-shaming—Baer uses erasure to blunt, reverse, or twist the original rhetorical intent.

Here, social media direct messages (DMs)—often dismissed as ephemeral digital noise—serve as fragmented archives of lived experience, documenting the intersections of public scrutiny, gendered labor, and intimate vulnerability in the social media age. By appropriating and redacting both hostile and supportive messages, Baer transforms them into curated life writing, where erasure becomes a form of autobiographical agency. As Andie Silva frames online interactions as traces of embodied existence, Baer treats DMs as raw material for self- representation: deleting others' words becomes a way to reclaim narrative control. Her erasure poems not only critique patriarchal and pandemic-era discourse but also archive her encounters with misogyny, caregiving, and survival, rendering the redacted page a palimpsest of lived reality. In this way, Baer redefines life writing as a subtractive practice, where the space between what is preserved and erased—like the silences in a diary—speak just as powerfully as the text itself, documenting a fractured yet insistent selfhood shaped by the digital public's gaze.

Baer's poem "Re: Comment Section under a Photo of a Tired Mother in Pandemic Times" uses such an approach, with the elaborate title itself prominently staging its aesthetic origins in digital communication. The original message, appearing on the left, compares the image of a mother during COVID-19 to iconic photos of mothers from the Great Depression.[22] Baer's erasure, composed more than a year into the pandemic, after multiple rounds of lockdowns and reopenings, counters these nostalgic evocations of maternal heroism. Her stripped-down poem reads:

> My small
> anguish
> the shape
> caregiving takes with fear and
> History.

More than the satisfying "gotcha" moment—described by Julia Spicher Kasdorf as a key feature of Baer's technique—the poem operates as a deliberate palimpsest. It speaks through what remains unsaid. The digital remains or marginalia speak entirely through absence. Visually dramatic, it is a concrete poem filled with redactions, holes, and omissions, rejecting the original text's uplifting tone and cohesive lines. The emphatic phrase—"YES SISTER I HEAR YOU" from the source text is erased. Solidarity, once claimed, is rendered absent—a casualty of the pandemic's capital-letter "History." The original ending—"Mothers are heroes"—is replaced by a single word: "History." Baer's method here becomes a means of asserting control over chaos. Her intervention is hybrid: not just verbal but also visual. Concrete poetry becomes a strategic form. The visual is not decorative—it asserts meaning. In this poem, once again, absence is the message. What once affirmed now fragments. Erasure becomes aesthetic form.

The centrality of erasure as an aesthetic focus continues into her third collection, *And Yet* (2022), sometimes appearing through strike-through, as in "Late

Summer ~~in a Global Pandemic~~,"[23] which crosses out "in a Global Pandemic." As with her black-out or redaction technique, the visible gesture suggests a tension between presence and absence, echoing what Mikhail Bakhtin described as a moment of crisis and identity liminality.[24] In these motherhood poems, the apparent erasure of the pandemic reflects how autobiographical poetry during the COVID-19 crisis became a site for negotiating the collapsing boundaries between private anguish and collective trauma. Baer's poetry reveals how autobiographical forms during the pandemic blurred the line between testimony and art. Its attention to the mundane does not diminish the scale of crisis but insists that global upheaval is felt most acutely in the fragments—like a scrap of paper scribbled by a child with an unanswered plea to his mother ("Can you jest be nice?"). Poetry here becomes neither refuge nor resolution, but a raw transcription of the body's struggle to endure.

"At the Covid Testing Clinic"

Only in her third collection, *And Yet* (2022)—published as COVID-19 began shifting to endemic status amid widespread booster vaccinations—does Baer name the virus directly, fuelled by her speaker's concerns about having become infected herself.

> I imagine the circumstances of my death—
> my husband bent and weeping, my children
> orphaned into little tremors of grief.
>
> Mask it or casket says the woman to my
> left. *Mother of four*, I text my husband.
> Too easy of a headline.
>
> They call my name, still alive for at
> least another hour. *Yes I'm here*, I say.
>
> I'm still here.[25]

Structured in two triplets, a couplet, and a final single line, this poem captures the tension between the speaker's awareness of the fragility of life and her continued existence amidst the uncertainty and fear of the COVID-19 pandemic. The speaker imagines her own death and the grief of her loved ones, while in the second triplet, the nearby woman's casual remark—"Mask it or casket"—underscores the looming presence of mortality. The second stanza acts as an imaginary obituary or epitaph headed "Mother of four," texted to her husband as executor, with a dose of self-critical gallows humor ("Too easy of a headline"). The couplet that follows these triplets returns the speaker to the present of the anonymous hospital staff to whom she is surrendering her fate.

The quiet declaration "I'm still here" in the last line becomes a poignant reminder of the uncertainty of pandemic survival, recalling philosopher Geoffrey Scarre's study "Killing Swiftly: The Experience of COVID-19 on the Elderly," which reflects on how the pandemic shattered complacent twenty-first-century beliefs in medicine's power to preserve life.[26] Though Scarre focuses primarily on the elderly, he also notes the suddenness and unexpectedness of COVID-related deaths among the middle-aged generations.[27] This unsettling awareness of mortality permeates Baer's poem. Even as the speaker situates herself in relation to her children and husband—naming those roles as central to her identity—she is alone in the clinic. While the speaker survives, the tone and structure carry elegiac weight, as her experience of pandemic-era social isolation and atomization reflects not just existential solitude but also the public health-induced collapse of communal life. Here the performance of poetic consciousness enacts life writing at the edge of death.

In the end, Kate Baer's poetry foregrounds the instability of selfhood amid crisis, treating identity as not only fluid but also socially, bodily, and digitally disrupted. As her work reveals, pandemic poetry straddles life writing and public discourse, using strategies of subtraction—alongside a play with presence and absence—to articulate the tension between private experience and collective disorientation. In this sense, erasure poetry functions as a mode of expressive endurance, collapsing boundaries between speaker and reader, individual and collective, within a post-digital space. As the examples discussed illustrate, Baer's use of poetic fragmentation techniques—gaps, silences, redaction, crossing-out—enacts a dual maneuver: it exposes the structural absences imposed by patriarchal power and pandemic precarity while simultaneously asserting agency through deliberate textual fragmentation. Her poetics generate a layered, discontinuous subjectivity—one that registers loss without surrendering narrative control.

In this way, the poem becomes a self-representational archive, simultaneously fragmented and insistent—a record not only of what is said but also of what is withheld, erased, or rewritten in dialogue with a reading public. Erasure poetry becomes, for Baer, a form of expressive survival—blurring the lines between witness and participant, poet and speaker, author and reader. Its viral circulation online, and its consolidation in bestselling print collections, recasts it as a medium of emotional communication, community formation, and memorialization during the pandemic.

Framing fragmented poetic utterance as both testimony and art—word and image—Baer's pandemic poetry affirms the continued relevance of lyric forms not as retreats from crisis, but as direct engagements with it. Poetry provides the aesthetic distance necessary to reflect on trauma without being overwhelmed by it. This essay also speaks to other contributions in this volume, including Brent Luvaas's and Chris Gilbert's respective chapters, whose lyrical pandemic photography and caricatured sketches become parallel practices of everyday witnessing. In this light, poetry functions not only as a record of survival but also as a form of life writing—transforming private anguish into a dispersed yet resonant collective voice, one that frames survival not as triumph but as the ongoing labor of living with loss, speaking through radical absence.

Notes

1 Kate Baer, "At the Covid Testing Clinic," in *And Yet* (Harper Perennial, 2022), 39.
2 Kitty O'Meara, *And the People Stayed Home* (New York: Simon and Schuster, 2020), 1–7.
3 Richard Hendrick, "Lockdown," *Ranch and Rural Living* 101, no. 9 (2020): 21.
4 See, for example, Tsitsi Ella Jaji, "Which Pandemic," *PMLA* 137, no. 1 (January 2022): 276–82, https://doi.org/10.1632/S0030812921000095.
5 Madalsa Mamgain and Zuivere Mamgain, *Get Lost Dirty Covid 19!* (Tellwell Talent [self-published], 2020), 57.
6 Quoted in Marcello Giovanelli, "Reading the Lockdown: Responding to Covid Poetry," *Journal of Poetry Therapy* 36, no. 3 (2020): 212.
7 Jeroen Dera, "Evaluating Poetry on COVID-19: Attitudes of Poetry Readers Toward Corona Poems," *Journal of Poetry Therapy* 34, no. 2 (2021): 77–94.
8 Daneshewar Sharma, "Reading and Rewriting Poetry on Life to Survive the COVID-19 Pandemic," *Journal of Poetry Therapy* 34, no. 2 (2021): 100.
9 Judith Blundell and Simon Poole, "Poetry in a Pandemic: Digital Shared Reading for Wellbeing," *Journal of Poetry Therapy* 36, no. 3 (2023): 198.
10 Ahron Friedberg, *Through a Screen Darkly: Psychoanalytic Reflections During the Pandemic*, ed. Sandra Sherman, 1st ed., vol. 1 (Routledge, 2021), https://doi.org/10.4324/9781003169994.
11 Kate Baer, "2020," in *What Kind of Woman* (Harper Perennial, 2020), 25.
12 Baer's critique of politics is echoed in many other poems including Rob D. Mitchell, "The Year of the 'Rona': An Uncontrolled Trial in Verse," *The Medical Journal of Australia* 213, no. 11 (2020): 524, critiquing the Australian governmental failures and the persistence of public suffering.
13 Kate Eichhorn, *Adjusted Margin: Xerography, Art, and Activism in the Late Twentieth Century* (Cambridge, MA: MIT Press, 2016).
14 Nathalie Cooke, "'Mi Rage': The Confessional Politics of Canadian Survivor Poetry," in *Confessional Politics: Women's Sexual Self-Representations in Life Writing and Popular Media*, ed. Irene Gammel (Carbondale: Southern Illinois University Press, 1999), 71.
15 Kate Baer, *What Kind of Woman* (Harper Perennial, 2020), 21.
16 Martina Topić, Marija Geiger Zeman, and Ivo Pilar, "Multiple Meanings of the Face Mask: Masking as the New Social Practice in the Context of Lockdown Creativity and Pandemic Chic," in *Creative Industries and Creative Economy*, Conference Proceedings (Zagreb: Vern University, 2021).
17 Sidonie Smith and Julia Watson, "Introduction," in *Interfaces: Women, Autobiography, Image, Performance* (University of Michigan Press, 2002), 10.
18 Spicher Kasdorf, "Kate Baer, *What Kind of Woman*, and Kate Baer, *I Hope This Finds You Well*, Book Review," *Journal of Mennonite Studies* 40, no. 2 (2022): 233.
19 Kate Baer, *I Hope This Finds You Well* (New York: Harper Perennial, 2021), x.
20 Baer, *I Hope*, xi.
21 This strategy is similar to Chinese author Fang Fang, *Wuhan Diary: Dispatches from a Quarantined City* (London: HarperCollins, 2020), which started online with daily blogs, responding to her audience's concerns; for more, see Irene Gammel and Jason Wang, "'Why Has the Outbreak Turned so Deadly?' Diary from a Quarantined City," in *Creative Resilience and COVID-19*, ed. Irene Gammel and Jason Wang (Routledge, 2022), 27–38.

22 Kate Baer, "Re: Comment Section Under a Photo of a Tired Mother in Pandemic Times," in *I Hope This Finds You Well* (New York: Harper Perennial, 2021), 60.
23 Kate Baer, "Late Summer ~~in a Global Pandemic~~," in *And Yet* (Harper Perennial, 2022), 6.
24 Baer's poem shares thematic ground with Cathy Fowley, "Grief in Times of Corona (Envoi)," *Qualitative Inquiry* 27, no. 7 (2021), which draws on Bakhtin through the metaphor of "bubbles" to express temporal and spatial fragmentation in crisis. Like Baer, Fowley contrasts COVID-19 grief with abstraction. Where Baer ends with "History," Fowley turns to numbers: "Bubble two—numbers: 25,489 cases in Ireland, 1,738 deaths, 112 days since I saw her, 47 days since I heard her voice." Fowley, "Grief in Times of Corona (Envoi)," 772.
25 Kate Baer, *And Yet* (Harper Perennial, 2022), 39.
26 Geoffrey Scarre, "Killing Swiftly: The Experience of COVID-19 on the Elderly," in *Creative Resilience and COVID-19: Figuring the Everyday in a Pandemic*, ed. Irene Gammel and Jason Wang (London: Routledge, 2022), 61.
27 Scarre, "Killing Swiftly," 64.

Bibliography

Baer, Kate. *And Yet*. New York: Harper Perennial, 2022.
Baer, Kate. *I Hope This Finds You Well*. New York: Harper Perennial, 2021.
Baer, Kate. *What Kind of Woman*. New York: Harper Perennial, 2020.
Baker, J. Scott. "Alone on Stage: How One LGBTIQ+ Educator Uses Poetic Performative Autoethnography for Social Change." *Journal of Education* 78 (2020): 24–42.
Blundell, Judith, and Simon Poole. "Poetry in a Pandemic: Digital Shared Reading for Wellbeing." *Journal of Poetry Therapy* 36, no. 3 (2023): 197–209.
Cooke, Nathalie. " 'Mi Rage': The Confessional Politics of Canadian Survivor Poetry." In *Confessional Politics: Women's Sexual Self-Representations in Life Writing and Popular Media*, edited by Irene Gammel, 63–80. Carbondale: Southern Illinois University Press, 1999.
Dera, Jeroen. "Evaluating Poetry on COVID-19: Attitudes of Poetry Readers Toward Corona Poems." *Journal of Poetry Therapy* 34, no. 2 (2021): 77–94.
Eichhorn, Kate. *Adjusted Margin: Xerography, Art, and Activism in the Late Twentieth Century*. Cambridge, MA: MIT Press, 2016.
Fowley, Cathy. "Grief in Times of Corona (Envoi)." *Qualitative Inquiry* 27, no. 7 (September 2020): 771–72.
Friedberg, Ahron. *Through a Screen Darkly: Psychoanalytic Reflections During the Pandemic*. Edited by Sandra Sherman. Routledge, 2021.
Gammel, Irene, and Jason Wang. " 'Why Has the Outbreak Turned so Deadly?' Diary from a Quarantined City." In *Creative Resilience and COVID-19*, edited by Irene Gammel and Jason Wang, 27–38. London: Routledge, 2022.
Giovanelli, Marcello. "Reading the Lockdown: Responding to Covid Poetry." *Journal of Poetry Therapy* 36, no. 3 (2022): 210–25.
Hendrick, Richard. "Lockdown." *Ranch and Rural Living* 101, no. 9 (2020): 21.
Mamgain, Madalsa, and Zuivere Mamgain. *Get Lost Dirty Covid 19!* Tellwell Talent (Self-Published), 2020.
McCullis, D. "Poetic Inquiry and Multidisciplinary Qualitative Research." *Journal of Poetry Therapy* 26, no. 2 (2013): 83–114.
Mitchell, Rob D. "The Year of the 'Rona': An Uncontrolled Trial in Verse." *Medical Journal of Australia* 213, no. 11 (December 2020): 524.
O'Meara, Kitty. *And the People Stayed Home*. New York: Simon and Schuster, 2020.
Satchidanandan, K., and Nishi Chawla, eds. *Singing in the Dark: A Global Anthology of Poetry Under Lockdown*. Vintage Books, Penguin Random House India, 2020.

Scarre, Geoffrey. "Killing Swiftly: The Experience of COVID-19 on the Elderly." In *Creative Resilience and COVID-19: Figuring the Everyday in a Pandemic*, edited by Irene Gammel and Jason Wang, 61–69. London: Routledge, 2022.

Sharma, D. "Reading and Rewriting Poetry on Life to Survive the COVID-19 Pandemic." *Journal of Poetry Therapy* 34, no. 2 (2021): 95–108.

Silva, Andie. "Reparatory Praxis." In *Feminist Digital Humanities: Theoretical, Social, and Material Engagements*, edited by Jacqueline Wernimont and Elizabeth Losh, 238–50. Minneapolis: University of Minnesota Press, 2018.

Smith, Sidonie, and Julia Watson. *Interfaces: Women, Autobiography, Image, Performance*. Ann Arbor: University of Michigan Press, 2002.

Spicher Kasdorf, Julia. "Kate Baer, *What Kind of Woman*, and Kate Baer, *I Hope This Finds You Well*, Book Review." *Journal of Mennonite Studies* 40, no. 2 (2022): 233–36.

Topić, Martina, Marija Geiger Zeman, and Ivo Pilar. "Multiple Meanings of the Face Mask: Masking as the New Social Practice in the Context of Lockdown Creativity and Pandemic Chic." In *Creative Industries and Creative Economy*, 132–45. Conference Proceedings. Zagreb: Vern University, 2021.

3

AFTERSHOCKS

"However Did I Pass the Time?" COVID-19 Autofiction as Trauma Narrative

Marjorie Worthington

Despite the widespread illness and death caused by COVID-19, there has yet to emerge a full cultural recognition of and reckoning with the trauma it wrought. This is particularly the case for those who did not become ill or lose loved ones to the disease but rather experienced the disease at some remove during the isolation period. For so many people, particularly white and affluent professional people, the lockdown was their primary experience of the COVID-19 era. The day- to-day monotony of working and schooling from home, the government-imposed distance from family and friends, the increased reliance on screens of various types rarely registered as acute suffering, particularly when the news contained near-constant images of widespread shortages, suffering, and death.

Nevertheless, these conditions have given rise to a distinct strain of Anglo-American autofiction in which narrators—often thinly veiled versions of their authors—grapple with the psychic fallout of lockdown life. Works such as Daisy Hildyard's *Emergency* (2022), Clare Pollard's *Delphi* (2022), Sigrid Nunez's *The Vulnerables* (2023), Chris Bachelder and Jennifer Habel's *Dayswork* (2023), and Louise Erdrich's *The Sentence* (2021) depict characters who remain COVID-free but endure a quieter, more ambiguous and long-term form of trauma. These autofictions usually do not confront the pandemic head-on but relegate it to the margins, echoing the formal strategies of trauma narrative, which often resists linearity, closure, and direct representation. This chapter argues that COVID autofiction turns to oblique narration and fragmented temporality not simply as aesthetic choices, but as necessary responses to the slow, suspended, and hard-to-grasp trauma of prolonged isolation. Ultimately, COVID-19 autofiction is an underexamined genre that directs the spotlight to the often unacknowledged—yet deeply pernicious—aftershocks of the pandemic.

DOI: 10.4324/9781003735595-5

Autofiction as Aftershock: Writing COVID-19 Through the Self

The term "autofiction" was coined in 1977 by French writer Serge Doubrovsky to describe his novel *Fils*: "Fiction, of facts and events strictly real, if you prefer, autofiction, where the language of adventure has been entrusted to the adventure of language in its total freedom."[1] As he later argued, autofiction refers to a mostly nonfictional, confessional form of writing. It depicts actual events but takes liberties with details and timelines. These narratives are both autobiographical and fictional: they are autofictional. In recent decades, autofiction has become virtually ubiquitous as a narrative mode and has been redefined many times.[2] In the definition I find most useful, the author-character diverges noticeably from the actual author; the events described may not accurately reflect extra-textual reality. Autofiction, then, provides insight into an author's persona by depicting that author in fictional, often ironic, ways. We see the author as through a glass, darkly.

Usually the autofictional author-character serves also as the protagonist and narrator, as is the case with most of the texts I will discuss. One notable exception is Louise Erdrich's *The Sentence,* in which a character named "Louise Erdrich" appears as a minor figure, described by the first-person narrator Tookie. The author-characters in autofictions like Daisy Hildyard's *Emergency* and Clare Pollard's *Delphi* are fictionalized versions of themselves, though the connection is often tenuous. *Delphi,* for example, features an unnamed narrator who resembles Clare Pollard, but also differs from her in significant ways. Each of these texts opens with a standard disclaimer—"any resemblance to actual persons living or dead . . . is entirely coincidental"[3]—yet the narrators clearly serve as fictionalized stand-ins for their authors, writing through the aftermath of COVID-19. Readers are invited to recognize both the personal and the fictional overlay. As Doubrovsky noted in an interview from 1997: "The meaning of one's life in certain ways escapes us, so we have to reinvent it in our writing, and that is what I personally call *autofiction.*"[4] This autofictional reinvention emerges as a useful way to make sense of life during the COVID-19 lockdown as it allows a search for meaning that unfolds through narrative experiments in self-representation. Much contemporary autofiction pursues this reinvention via formal experimentation.

Novels like Ben Lerner's *10:04* (2014), Arthur Phillips's *The Tragedy of Arthur* (2011), and Bret Easton Ellis's *Lunar Park* (2005) and *The Shards* (2023) place real-life author-characters in overtly fictional situations. The name connection between author and protagonist highlights the friction between text and real life. In contrast, COVID autofiction tends to use unnamed narrators, making the connection implicit. This shift in strategy reflects not just a stylistic choice but also a deeper thematic kinship with what has come to be termed "trauma narrative."

Richard McNally defines trauma as involving "an objectively defined event, the person's subjective interpretation of its meaning, and the person's emotional reaction to it," stressing that trauma is shaped by an individual or cultural reaction to the event itself. Trauma scholar Cathy Caruth points out that trauma "is not assimilated or experienced fully at the time, but only belatedly,"[5] which is why survivors often process trauma through repeated returns. In this way, both individual and cultural traumas are shaped by storytelling, or—as Shoshana Felman argues—that for traumatic memory to lose its grip, "a therapeutic process—a process of constructing a narrative, of reconstructing a history and essentially, of *re-externalizing the event*—has to be set in motion."[6] Roger Luckhurst observes that trauma "issues a challenge to the capacities of narrative knowledge," generating what he calls "the manic production of retrospective narratives that seek to explicate the trauma."[7]

In other words, "trauma narrative" transforms traumatic memory into narrative memory.[8] It often rejects traditional linear structure in favor of formal strategies that echo trauma's disorienting effects. Michelle Balaev refers to "narrative dissociation"—where repetition and negation disrupt perception[9]—and Laurence Kirmayer notes that amnesia or repression may also be rendered narratively.[10] Anne Whitehead identifies recurring stylistic features: "intertextuality, repetition and a dispersed or fragmented narrative voice."[11] For Luckhurst, trauma narratives are "experimental, fragmented . . . and suspicious of familiar representational and narrative conventions."[12] Laurie Vickroy emphasizes how they "internalize the rhythms, processes and uncertainties of traumatic experience."[13] COVID-19 autofictions inhabit this space. In both form and content, these texts blur the boundary between personal reflection and narrative disruption.

They invent meaning amid uncertainty, revisiting the self not to stabilize identity, but to record its trembling. COVID-19 autofictions not only reinvent the self but they also register a broader collective rupture—less from a single dramatic event than from the slow, destabilizing effects of lockdown: a private experience shared across cultures.

The COVID-19 virus took millions of lives and often left survivors with lasting illness; it put enormous stress on health care systems, hospitals, and healthcare workers. In other words, the traumatic aspect of the disease itself is evident. Less visible at the time was the psychological toll of lockdown on those able to isolate. True, these people were more protected from the virus, yet with hindsight, the deleterious results of isolation are coming into sharper focus.[14] To paraphrase Cathy Caruth, the traumatic meaning of that COVID lockdown could not be fully assimilated while it was happening. And while the COVID-19 disease is still with us, the lockdown has ended, allowing us to look back and try to "possess" it—to integrate it into our both our self-definition and cultural zeitgeist. COVID-19 autofiction participates in this effort, shaping personal experience into a form that might be shared and understood.

Often building upon discussions of literary reactions to the 1918 so-called Spanish Flu Epidemic,[15] scholars like Rocio Palomeque Recio, drawing from Gilad Hirschberger, frame "the recent global pandemic and its attached restrictions of free movement for a large part of the world's population as a collective trauma, bringing with it a crisis of meaning and a reconstruction of social categories."[16]

Hirschberger defines "collective trauma" as "the psychological reactions to a traumatic event that affects an entire society." He continues:

> It suggests that the tragedy is represented in the collective memory of the group, and like all forms of memory it comprises not only a reproduction of the events, but also an ongoing reconstruction of the trauma in an attempt to make sense of it.[17]

COVID-19 narratives—notably autofiction—contribute to that reconstruction. Some chronicle individual experience, others offer oblique mediations on loss, isolation, and social rupture—but all are helping shape a shared cultural memory of that time.

COVID Autofiction in Daisy Hildyard's *Emergency* and Sigrid Nunez's *The Vulnerables*

In contrast to narratives about direct experience with the COVID-19 virus, most of the COVID- 19 autofiction I have encountered focuses primarily on the lockdown rather than the disease and tends to place the ensuing crisis on the narrative's periphery. These works avoid lengthy, unwavering focus on the realities of illness or confinement; instead, they provide a flash of the moment before shifting attention away from it—as if recoiling from a too-bright object. Hoyt Long et al. found something similar in their study of personal social media narratives about the COVID-19-lockdown: "After the initial traumatic shock of the virus outbreak and subsequent containment measures, these writers gradually came to internalize the pandemic as a background presence rather than an explicit fact."[18] Two elements are likely at play here: the lockdown is both somewhat boring to depict and also traumatic—something these writers had not yet fully assimilated. On a larger scale, in this post-lockdown period, the experience of COVID-19-era isolation seems to have disappeared into what Catherine Belling calls "collective amnesia." Belling, writing about fiction from the 1918 flu era, makes a point that could easily apply to the COVID-19 texts I discuss here: "the fiction tends to replicate some of the pandemic's resistance to being recalled and recounted."[19] The narrative strategies of autofiction serve as excellent vehicles for portraying this resistance.

Because autofiction purports to depict the author's actual experience while flagrantly departing into fiction, it evokes the author-character yet simultaneously constructs a separation between the author and the narrator. In other words, the autofiction both is and is *not* an accurate representation of its author's life. This strategy becomes useful in COVID-19 autofiction, allowing the author to seem to represent their own experience of lockdown while also avoiding direct representation. In this way, the narrator can portray the author's traumatic experience without completely implicating the author and their life.

In her discussion of Kurt Vonnegut's 1969 novel *Slaughterhouse-Five*, Susanne Vees- Gulani describes the effect of having narrator of the novel be a fictionalized version of Vonnegut himself: "Removing himself from the factual to the fictional plane by creating the narrator allows Vonnegut a degree of distance from himself and his experiences."[20] In autofictional fashion, the narrator of *Slaughterhouse-Five* both is and is not Vonnegut himself. The distance between author and narrator provides the space necessary for Vonnegut to narrativize the trauma of the 1945 firebombing of Dresden, which the 22-year-old Vonnegut was involved in as a prisoner of war. In the case of COVID-19 autofiction, such distancing becomes a way to narrate the trauma of lockdown.

A primary characteristic of COVID-19 autofiction, then, is its resistance to depicting the pandemic directly—instead performing a kind of talking around the crisis. These works are ostensibly *about* the COVID-19 era, but often mention it only in passing. In an interview, Daisy Hildyard, author of *Emergency*, describes a complex relationship to autofiction: it was both a genre she admired and one she deliberately resisted. "I read a lot of autofiction because I like a feeling of plainness in a story," she explains, appreciating its pared-down aesthetic.[21] At the same time, she was uneasy with a recurring structure in the genre: books that "moved digressively, from one subject to another, via associations in the author-narrator's memory or consciousness." What troubled her was how this inward-looking mode seemed to distort the world outside the self, rendering it "like this half-chewed substance, always pushed through the digestive system of the narrator's thoughts." Hildyard's novel tries to break from that pattern. Rather than filtering everything through a single perspective, *Emergency* aims to depict "life pouring or rushing, with many different beings colliding with one another, stories converging and diverging."

Emergency employs several of the narrative strategies that characterize trauma narrative, including repression and a dispersed or fragmented voice. It consists mostly of ruminations on the unnamed narrator's rural Yorkshire childhood, punctuated by fleeting accounts of her present-day lockdown life in London. The comparison is stark between her earlier experiences—roaming the countryside, building gardens, caring for livestock—and her present, which goes unnamed until page 41: "It's April and I'm not allowed to leave the house more than once a day." She elaborates: "I haven't been outside now for sixteen days. I have been instructed to shelter in place."[22] The narrator briefly describes writing, spying through windows at neighbors she doesn't know, tracking ants on her houseplants. But the narrative quickly shifts again into memories of childhood—especially memories of being outdoors.

On a video call during lockdown, a friend tells her that her boyfriend has left her and their two children, as pandemic stress worsened their relationship. The narrator almost immediately shifts to describing helping a childhood neighbor on his farm—as though she can only tolerate brief encounters with the present before retreating back into the past. The isolation of her life creates a strange distance from COVID: "I haven't felt that the disease out there in the world is real," she notes, even while suspecting her neighbor may have caught it.[23] While the titular emergency feels remote—trauma lying more in the fear and solipsism of isolation, COVID-19 being slow-moving and cumulative, not sudden in its impact—the autofiction makes readers consider the idea of an emergency, whose very etymology is linked to the verb *emerge* in the sense of *emerging suddenly*. And while the narrator is aware that people handle grief in different ways—some taking time to mourn and process their emotions, while others "keep busy"—whether through fitness routines, social groups, demanding work schedules, or tending to their gardens,[24] much of the novel focuses on "keeping busy," or skirting around the present.

Indeed, the narrator is so absorbed in being "busy" that she misses the start of a real emergency that closes this novel—a fire just outside her home, "the homes of my neighbors, in the building opposite, had disappeared inside the blaze."[25] The crisis hits home and demands attention, with neighbors gathering in the street, interacting in ways they had not done for months—and the narrator no longer able to withdraw from the trauma of the present. In this moment, *Emergency* delivers a jolt—a turning point that resists the limits of what autofiction can and cannot do: it begins in the genre's familiar mode of introspection and digression but ends by challenging that inwardness—by forcing the narrator, and the reader, outward.

A similar form of isolation faces the unnamed narrator of Sigrid Nunez's 2023 autofiction novel *The Vulnerables*, set not in London but New York. The title marks her status—being well over 65 and thus "vulnerable" to COVID-19—though her economic privilege shields her from material risk. Wealthy friends, having decamped to their country home, ask her stay in their upscale apartment to care for their parrot, Eureka. Like the narrator of *Emergency*, Nunez's narrator is less affected by the illness than by the psychic toll of isolation. Her trauma stems from restrictions, not illness. She registers her privilege with self-ironic awareness that is typical of autofiction: "What lockdown? went the viral tweet," she quotes, describing the pandemic as "the middle class hiding while working-class people bring them things." Another version: "white people hiding while Black and brown people bring them things."[26] Yet even in safety, the stillness wears on her: "Looking back, I would always wonder: However did I pass the time?" Her answer—"I read a lot of news, but other reading—reading for pleasure—had become too hard"[27]—speaks to the cognitive fragmentation experienced by many. Even literature, the traditional refuge, offers no reprieve: "I found myself tuning out so often that I lost the thread of the story."[28]

While these elements echo other COVID-19 novels, what distinguishes *The Vulnerables*—and makes it central to my study of COVID-19 autofiction—is its explicit defense of the form. Without using the word "autofiction," Nunez critiques the conventional novel's waning relevance: "The traditional novel has lost its place as the major genre of our time," she writes, asserting that "No matter how imaginative, it seems to lack originality."[29] She turns instead to a literature grounded in personal narrative, evoking a new "literature of personal history and reflection:

direct, authentic, scrupulous about fact."[30] This is autofiction as a deliberate counter to "our own dark anti-truth times,"[31] where storytelling becomes a tool of distortion, of half-truths and untruths. Against a landscape of discursive excess, her slim, elliptical narrative attempts something bold: to restore literature's truth-value by exposing its own fragilities.

In this way, *The Vulnerables* not only exemplifies but also actively theorizes autofiction as a form uniquely suited to the pandemic era—an era defined by unreliable narratives, fractured attention, and blurred boundaries between public crisis and private response. Nunez's narrator is attuned to her own unreliability, haunted by intrusive thoughts, obsessively replaying "every bad or stupid thing I'd ever said or done."[32] She confronts the dilemma of how much to reveal, asking: "to describe, or not to describe, those thoughts?"[33] This is the ethical tension at the heart of autofiction: the demand to tell the truth, while knowing the self is always a precarious and unstable witness. Her acknowledgment of cognitive distortion—catastrophizing, memory gaps, nightmarish recall—does not discredit her narrative but rather strengthens it. Autofiction here functions as a genre and, more pressingly, as a method of survival: truth-telling that wrestles with its own complexity.

Author as Oracle: Autofictional Turns in *Dayswork* and *Delphi*

While *Emergency* and *The Vulnerables* depict the isolation wrought by lockdown in order to reflect upon how COVID-19 shapes autofiction itself, Chris Bachelder and Jennifer Habel's *Dayswork* (2022) and Clare Pollard's *Delphi* (2023) focus on the pressure that lockdown put on marriages and families, but take similar tacks in their distracted portrayals of life during COVID-19. *Dayswork* centers around a family of four living in Cincinnati during lockdown. Although written by both Bachelder and Habel, the single unnamed narrator is the wife,[34] whose description of day-to-day struggles with COVID-19 realities is overshadowed by her researched explorations into the lives and marriages of Nathanial Hawthorne, Robert Lowell, Elizabeth Hardwick, Sylvia Plath, and, primarily, Herman Melville. The novel provides fleeting glimpses of family life during lockdown: the children do Zoom school and the husband works from home—eventually contracting COVID-19 and quarantining in their basement. However, the bulk of the book consists of snippets of factual information about and quotations from the writers, about whom the narrator becomes increasingly obsessed. Over the course of the text, a narrative emerges about Melville's life, his relationship with Nathaniel Hawthorne, and, to a lesser extent, a narrative about other writers who admired Melville, most notably the married poets Robert Lowell and Elizabeth Hardwick.

It is unclear how or why this research began, but the narrator's focus on Melville clearly stems from an admiration of his work, and the text is replete with quotations praising him from writers and scholars across time. Her husband jokes that, during the pandemic, she has "contracted Melville,"[35] as the post-it notes containing these quotations flutter around the house, sticking out of her books and getting lost in their bedsheets. These tidbits together paint a picture of Melville's career, early struggles, successes and failures, friendships, and marriage. Indeed, the text is more about Melville and other writers than it is about the author and her family. Just as the other works I have discussed only tangentially address the pandemic, *Dayswork* offers fleeting scenes of the family's current living circumstances and furtive mentions of previous marital problems, referred to as "The Bad Time," when her husband "went far away" in their small house: "I'm *right here*, he would say, wrongly."[36] Directly after this personal note, the narrator launches into a lengthy discussion of the average life spans of Emily Dickinson, Byron and Melville. The narrator's life—painful, joyful, or mundane—is parceled out in tiny increments surrounded by seemingly random literary facts.

As the work progresses, however, the pattern becomes clear: Melville's career—like Tolstoy's and Lowell's—was built on the labor of their wives. Lizzie Melville wrote of "romantic occupations"—cleaning his study, filling his inkwell, copying manuscripts, and reading to him at night.[37] Sophia Tolstoy copied *War and Peace* seven times by candlelight.[38] For over two decades, Elizabeth Hardwick managed Lowell's life while enduring his public infidelities.[39] These glimpses into their marriages reveal that literary "greatness" often relied on women's unacknowledged work. The implication is that, throughout literary history, men are enabled to write because the women in their lives do the day's work, the *Dayswork.* The narrator begins to question the authorial myths of greatness. Admiring Lowell becomes more difficult upon learning he broke his first wife's nose. Melville, too, seems less admirable when evidence suggests he may have abused his wife. Scholars attempt to excuse these men, but the narrator—and readers—find it harder to do so. Their genius looks smaller once we see whose shoulders it stood upon.

We get brief hints that the narrator's marriage bears similar strains exacerbated by the lockdown stresses. To be clear, no physical or verbal abuse is depicted, but the narrator carries much of the husband's weight. Early in their marriage, "many nights our conversations turned tense—Whatever our topic, our topic was in fact the terms of our new marriage."[40] Later: "During the Bad Time my husband and I disagreed about moving to another state. To this one. I lost."[41] When her husband quarantines in the basement, the narrator runs the household and cares for him: her husband "requires a lot, but he doesn't ask for much."[42] These sentiments, while telling, are scattered and treated like literary tidbits rather than stark reflections of their marriage. *Dayswork* acts as a camera obscura through which we glimpse the pressure COVID-19 lockdown placed on the couple's marriage without explicit and painful description. The text echoes Breanne Fahs's account of the "grotesque inequalities in gendered household labor" laid bare by COVID-19, which brought "regressive changes" that disproportionately burdened women—intensifying domestic, emotional, sexual, parental, and educational labor, while merging paid work with home life and increasing exposure to domestic violence.[43] These lives unfold through a literary lens, their stories fragmented and nonlinear, marked by an offhanded tone characteristic of trauma narratives. Writing the past becomes a way to cope with the present, constructing a narrative of survival.

Rather than focus on the past, Clare Pollard's *Delphi* (2023) features a narrator who researches ways of predicting the future. The narrator, a classicist and translator (like Pollard), lives in London with her husband and 10-year-old son Xander. Although much of the text describes oracular traditions and modes of fortune telling, it opens with the narrator declaring: "I am sick of the future," insisting: "I don't want anything to do with it; don't want it near me."[44] This sentiment is understandable for someone living and raising a family in London's lockdown, especially someone who worries aloud about her sensitive, highly allergic son: "*I don't know if my son will even live to middle age.*"[45] It is hard to look forward when the present is dangerous, uncertain, and monotonous, but even before the pandemic, she felt: "It is not going to get better than this. I will age and diminish. And the world, too, diminishes." She asks: "Why do I want to have an affair, leave, quit my job, anything? Because otherwise nothing will ever happen again."[46] When the virus began spreading, "it's disappointing, but in a way I am also thrilled because something is happening. Everyone is thrilled, actually! We are so bored of our unreal lives it is a change, at least; it is history happening."[47]

Indeed, the pandemic triggered a rupture in temporality, heightening the narrator's historical consciousness, in turn, prompting the narrator to shift toward magical thinking to regain agency, with divination taking center stage—reflected in the novel's title, *Delphi*. Amid the boredom of their unreal lives during the long pandemic, the narrator becomes obsessed with researching soothsaying traditions—ancient oracles, the zodiac, tarot, palm reading, and the I Ching—seeking ways to tell the future. She claims this research is for her next book about "prophecy in the ancient world,"[48] but her interest broadens to examples worldwide and across time. Like in *Dayswork*, scenes from her present life are interwoven with deep dives into esoteric traditions, with research becoming both obsession and refuge. Though she admits she doesn't truly believe in these fortune-telling methods, she consults them compulsively: "I feel this abject, poisonous need to know what's next."[49] That need grows as her marriage frays, her son's mental health declines, and COVID enters their family, likely killing their great-grandmother.

During a psychic reading, "Rae turns over—of course she does—the Ten of Cups. The rainbow, the loving couple, the happy children. I flinch as though at the spring of a trap. 'Domestic bliss,' she says. 'Lucky you.'"[50] The prediction comes true, but at a cost: her son attempts suicide, survives, and her marriage stabilizes in the aftermath. The novel ends with her holding her son's hand, telling him the story of the Sibylline Books. It is a fragile image of domestic unity, shadowed by trauma and still haunted by the urge to foresee. *Delphi* suggests that the true impact of the pandemic may defy direct depiction—yet in a single moment, its force can snap into focus. Though the narrator longs for the future, in the end, it is the present that demands her attention. Ultimately, *Delphi*'s use of oracular practices being anchored in temporality and a focus on the future underscores how autofiction works toward repair—not by direct depiction but by creating decipherable patterns and grounding experience within time.

Autofiction's Afterlife—Redux

As I conclude my study of autofiction in COVID-19 life writing, I turn to one final novel that makes its author a character. Louise Erdrich's *The Sentence* (2021) shares with the other texts an indirect portrayal of the author's COVID-19 experience, yet differs by rendering "Louise," the author-character, in the third person rather than the first. Unlike most autofiction, *The Sentence* is narrated not by an authorial avatar but by Tookie, a Native American bibliophile who, after a stint in prison, finds work at Birchbark Books in Minneapolis—the real-life bookstore owned by Erdrich herself. Nevertheless, even though Tookie's husband contracts and nearly dies of COVID-19—making *The Sentence* more explicit about the disease than other works discussed here—as in the previous works, the author-character "Louise" appears only peripherally. As Tookie observes, "The life of the writer cannot help but haunt the narrative."[51] "Louise" hovers on margins, not central to the plot but still present as an autofictional force. When the bookstore is forced to close in the early days of the lockdown, the loss hits differently for each character. For temporarily Tookie, it means unemployment; for "Louise," it is a deeper existential blow:

> She had this weird sense of destiny about the store. It was more than a place, it was a nexus, a mission, a work of art, a calling, a sacred craziness, a slice of eccentricity, a collection of good people who shifted and rearranged but cared deeply about the same one thing—books.[52]

When bookselling is deemed essential and the store partially reopens, "Louise" is "jubilant": "It means bookstores are deemed *essential* businesses, Tookie."[53] The image of bookselling as "essential" crystallizes how autofiction makes the ordinary profound—revealing how stories, like books, become lifelines in a crisis, grounding fragmented experience and affirming shared human resilience.

This tension—the author both present and peripheral—captures autofiction's complex negotiation between presence and absence, showing how COVID-19 life writing resists straightforward representation, its trauma haunting the narrative's margins. In the end, we return to the idea of autofiction as registering the aftershock of the pandemic obliquely. Autofiction's distinctive power during the COVID-19 pandemic lies in its capacity to register a trauma that is both diffuse and deferred. Rather than documenting illness, these narratives trace the atmospheric damage of disrupted time, social estrangement, and the slow disintegration of the self. By filtering lockdown life through fictionalized selves, autofiction offers a space in which meaning can be provisionally shaped, deferred, or disavowed altogether. The narrators in texts like *Delphi* and *Emergency* are not heroic survivors or public witnesses; they are porous figures, shaped by what they cannot fully comprehend or directly narrate. This formal obliqueness—unnamed narrators, non-linear timelines, fragmented perspectives—is not a failure to address the pandemic but a deliberate way of engaging with a trauma that lacks the spectacle or narrative resolution traditionally associated with catastrophe. Autofiction thus emerges as a particularly apt genre for capturing the slow violence of pandemic time and its unspoken psychological aftermath. As COVID-19 recedes from immediate public discourse, autofiction continues to bear its imprint—not as historical documentation but as aftershock.

These autofictions do not aim to preserve a factual record but rather to convey the subjective disorientation of life during and after lockdown. Triggered by rupture in ordinary temporality, the pandemic, even in its nominal "post" phase, remains ambient in these texts—an absent presence that shapes tone, form, and consciousness. In making room for ambiguity, contradiction, and reinvention, COVID autofiction provides an enduring model for how literature can respond to collective trauma without subsuming it into a tidy narrative. It reminds us that life writing is not always about clarity or confession; sometimes it is about registering the world sideways, through a glass, darkly.

Notes

1 Serge Doubrovsky, "Autofiction," *Autofiction* 1 (2013): i.
2 I provide a historical overview of these various definitions in my book *The Story of "Me": Contemporary American Autofiction* (University of Nebraska Press, 2018).
3 Sigrid Nunez, *The Vulnerables* (New York: Riverhead Books, 2023), i. The disclaimer in *The Sentence* departs somewhat from the standard language by saying, "Any resemblance to actual events, locales, organizations, or persons, living or dead, is entirely coincidental. Except for the dictionary and the ghost." Louise Erdrich, *The Sentence* (New York: HarperCollins, 2021).
4 Roger Célestin, "Interview with Serge Doubrovsky: Autofiction and Beyond," *Journal of the Twentieth Century/Contemporary French Studies* 1, no. 2 (2001): 400.
5 Cathy Caruth, ed., *Trauma: Explorations in Memory* (Baltimore: Johns Hopkins University Press, 1995), 4.
6 Shoshana Felman and Dori Laub, *Testimony: Crises of Witnessing in Literature, Psychoanalysis, and History* (New York: Routledge, 1991), 69.
7 Roger Luckhurst, *The Trauma Question* (New York: Routledge, 2008), 79.
8 Anne Whitehead, *Trauma Fiction* (Edinburgh: Edinburgh University Press, 2004), 140.
9 Michelle Balaev, *The Nature of Trauma in American Novels* (Evanston, IL: Northwestern University Press, 2012), xvi.
10 Laurence Kirmayer, "Landscapes of Memory: Trauma, Narrative, and Dissociation," in *Tense Past: Cultural Essays in Trauma and Memory*, ed. Paul Antze and Michael Lambek (New York: Routledge, 1996), 180.
11 Whitehead, *Trauma Fiction*, 84.
12 Luckhurst, *The Trauma Question*, 81.
13 Laurie Vickroy, *Trauma and Survival in Contemporary Fiction* (Charlottesville: University of Virginia Press, 2002), 3.
14 An article from the National Institutes of Health states: "Many people are likely to develop a wide range of mental health issues due to being quarantined, and/or as a result of job loss, such as low mood, insomnia, irritability, depression and posttraumatic

stress disorder." Michaéla C. Schippers, "For the Greater Good? The Devastating Ripple Effects of the COVID-19 Crisis," *Frontiers in Psychology* 11 (2020): 5.

15 The so-called Spanish Flu was an outbreak of an H1N1 virus that, between 1918 and 1920, killed 657,000 people in the United States and more than 50 million people worldwide. Although the first known case was traced to Kansas, it became known as the "Spanish Flu" because World War I censorship standards kept the press in many countries from reporting on the disease; because Spain was not involved in the war, the Spanish press reported freely about the disease, giving the international impression that it had begun and was largely focused in Spain.

16 Rocio Palomeque Recio, "Postfeminist Performance of Domesticity and Motherhood During the COVID-19 Global Lockdown: The Case of Chiara Ferragni," *Feminist Media Studies* 22, no. 3 (2020): 658–59.

17 Gilad Hirschberger, "Collective Trauma and the Social Construction of Meaning," *Frontiers in Psychology* 9 (2018): 1.

18 Hoyt Long, Richard Jean So, and Kaitlyn Todd, "#COVID, Crisis, and the Search for Story in the Platform Age," *Critical Inquiry* 49, no. 4 (2023): 548–49.

19 Catherine Belling, "Overwhelming the Medium: Fiction and the Trauma of Pandemic Influenza in 1918," *Literature and Medicine* 28, no. 1 (2009): 59.

20 Susanne Vees-Gulani, "Diagnosing Billy Pilgrim: A Psychiatric Approach to Kurt Vonnegut's *Slaughterhouse-Five*," *Critique* 44, no. 2 (2003): 182.

21 Helen Whybrow and Daisy Hildyard, "Slow Violence: An Interview with Daisy Hildyard," *Orion Magazine*, December 6, 2022, https://orionmagazine.org/article/emergency-daisy-hildyard-interview-2022/. The quotations in the rest of this paragraph are from the same interview and source.

22 Daisy Hildyard, *Emergency* (New York: Astra House, 2022), 41.

23 Hildyard, *Emergency*, 153.

24 Hildyard, *Emergency*, 43.

25 Hildyard, *Emergency*, 210–11.

26 Nunez, *The Vulnerables*, 98.

27 Nunez, *The Vulnerables*, 174.

28 Nunez, *The Vulnerables*, 174.

29 Dwight Garner, "In the Early Days of Lockdown, a Writer Considers a Perplexing Age," *The New York Times*, October 30, 2023. The quotations in the rest of this paragraph are from the same interview and source.

30 Nunez quoted in Garner, "Early Days of Lockdown."

31 Nunez, *The Vulnerables*, 227.

32 Nunez, *The Vulnerables*, 175.

33 Nunez, *The Vulnerables*, 174.

34 That the narrator is a characterized version of Jennifer Habel is implied when we are told that the narrator's husband's name is "Chris" (215). This onomastic connection suggests an identity between author and character that is disputed by the disclaimer at the beginning of the text: "*Dayswork* is a novel. Apart from the well-known actual people, historical events, and locales that figure in the narrative, characters and incidents are the products of the authors' imaginations or are used fictitiously" (Bachelder and Habel). The resultant ambiguity about whether the character does or does not represent the author is part of the autofictional project. Chris Bachelder and Jennifer Habel, *Dayswork* (New York: W.W. Norton & Co., Inc., 2023), 215, i.

35 Bachelder and Habel, *Dayswork*, 3.

36 Bachelder and Habel, *Dayswork*, 29.

37 Bachelder and Habel, *Dayswork*, 88.

38 Bachelder and Habel, *Dayswork*, 71.

39 Bachelder and Habel, *Dayswork*, 93.

40 Bachelder and Habel, *Dayswork*, 82.

41 Bachelder and Habel, *Dayswork*, 114.
42 Bachelder and Habel, *Dayswork*, 201.
43 Breanne Fahs, "'He's Thinking About Sex, I'm Thinking About Survival': Women's Sexual, Domestic, and Emotional Labor During the COVID-19 Pandemic," in *Creative Resilience and COVID-19: Figuring the Everyday in a Pandemic*, ed. Irene Gammel and Jason Wang (London: Routledge, 2022), 70.
44 Clare Pollard, *Delphi* (New York: Simon & Schuster, 2022), 1.
45 Pollard, *Delphi*, 1.
46 Pollard, *Delphi*, 15–16.
47 Pollard, *Delphi*, 18.
48 Pollard, *Delphi*, 7.
49 Pollard, *Delphi*, 176.
50 Pollard, *Delphi*, 178–79.
51 Erdrich, *The Sentence*, 164.
52 Erdrich, *The Sentence*, 189.
53 Erdrich, *The Sentence*, 190.

Bibliography

Bachelder, Chris, and Jennifer Habel. *Dayswork*. New York: W.W. Norton & Co., Inc., 2023.

Balaev, Michelle. *The Nature of Trauma in American Novels*. Evanston, IL: Northwestern University Press, 2012.

Belling, Catherine. "Overwhelming the Medium: Fiction and the Trauma of Pandemic Influenza in 1918." *Literature and Medicine* 28, no. 1 (2009): 55–81. https://doi.org/10.1353/lm.0.0046.

Caruth, Cathy, ed. *Trauma: Explorations in Memory*. Baltimore: Johns Hopkins University Press, 1995.

Célestin, Roger. "Interview with Serge Doubrovsky: Autofiction and Beyond." *Journal of the Twentieth Century/Contemporary French Studies* 1, no. 2 (2001): 397–405.

Dickinson, Emily. "Tell All the Truth but Tell It Slant (1263)." In *The Poems of Emily Dickinson: Reading Edition*, edited by R.W. Franklin. Cambridge, MA: The Belknap Press of Harvard University Press, 1998.

Doubrovsky, Serge. "Autofiction." *Auto/Fiction* 1 (2013): i–ii.

Erdrich, Louise. *The Sentence*. New York: HarperCollins, 2021.

Fahs, Breanne. "'He's Thinking About Sex, I'm Thinking About Survival': Women's Sexual, Domestic, and Emotional Labor During the COVID-19 Pandemic." In *Creative Resilience and COVID-19: Figuring the Everyday in a Pandemic*, edited by Irene Gammel and Jason Wang, 70–81. London: Routledge, 2022.

Felman, Shoshana, and Dori Laub. *Testimony: Crises of Witnessing in Literature, Psychoanalysis, and History*. New York: Routledge, 1991.

Hildyard, Daisy. *Emergency*. New York: Astra House, 2022.

Hirschberger, Gilad. "Collective Trauma and the Social Construction of Meaning." *Frontiers in Psychology* 9 (2018): 1–14. https://doi.org/10.3389/fpsyg.2018.01441.

Kirmayer, Laurence. "Landscapes of Memory: Trauma, Narrative, and Dissociation." In *Tense Past: Cultural Essays in Trauma and Memory*, edited by Paul Antze and Michael Lambek, 173–98. New York: Routledge, 1996.

Long, Hoyt, Richard Jean So, and Kaitlyn Todd. "#COVID, Crisis, and the Search for Story in the Platform Age." *Critical Inquiry* 49, no. 4 (2023): 530–56. https://doi.org/10.1086/725059.

Luckhurst, Roger. *The Trauma Question*. New York: Routledge, 2008.

McNally, Richard. *Remembering Trauma*. Cambridge, MA: Belknap, 2003.

Nunez, Sigrid. *The Vulnerables*. New York: Riverhead Books, 2023.

Palomeque Recio, Rocio. "Postfeminist Performance of Domesticity and Motherhood During the COVID-19 Global Lockdown: The Case of Chiara Ferragni." *Feminist Media Studies* 22, no. 3 (2020): 657–78. https://doi.org/10.1080/14680777.2020.1830147.

Pollard, Clare. *Delphi*. New York: Simon & Schuster, 2022.

Schippers, Michaéla C. "For the Greater Good? The Devastating Ripple Effects of the COVID-19 Crisis." *Frontiers in Psychology* 11 (2020): 1–13. https://doi.org/10.3389/Fpsyg.2020.577740.

Vees-Gulani, Susanne. "Diagnosing Billy Pilgrim: A Psychiatric Approach to Kurt Vonnegut's *Slaughterhouse-Five*." *Critique* 44, no. 2 (2003): 175–84.

Versluys, Kristiaan. *Out of the Blue: September 11 and the Novel*. New York: Columbia University Press, 2009.

Vickroy, Laurie. *Trauma and Survival in Contemporary Fiction*. Charlottesville: University of Virginia Press, 2002.

Whitehead, Anne. *Trauma Fiction*. Edinburgh: Edinburgh University Press, 2004.

4

BEYOND *WUHAN DIARY*

Rethinking Autobiographical Norms Amid COVID-19

Marjorie Dryburgh

In both my teaching and research, I'm drawn to the challenge of working with fragmentary, partial, or contradictory sources. Whether guiding students through China's modern history or examining its inter-war years, I focus on how we locate, assess, and interpret imperfect evidence with rigor and openness. This approach demands attention to voices that might otherwise be silenced. It shapes my work on autobiographical writing from China during the COVID-19 pandemic, when a surge of diaries, memoirs, and digital testimonies emerged amid lockdown, uncertainty, and grief. These texts offer intimate glimpses of life under state control and collective trauma but also pose difficult questions: What is said—and what remains unspoken? What gets preserved, published, or erased? As these personal stories were eagerly consumed for their assumed immediacy and authenticity, they were also scrutinized for breaches—had writers behaved "properly" during lockdown? Had they respected norms of self-narrative, including standards of evidence, self-presentation, and the uses of their stories?

In reading these accounts, I'm interested not only in what they reveal about the pandemic but also in how they push us to rethink the fragile, difficult work of telling one's own story under constraint. Life writing scholars Sidonie Smith and Julia Watson note that such writing often "speaks in silences, in absences, in what cannot be said," a point echoed in the COVID-19 poetry discussed by Irene Gammel and Jason Wang, who describe it as marked by "radical absence" (see Chapter 2). More specifically, this chapter engages with life writing theorist Paul John Eakin's concept of "autobiographical living"—the ongoing internal process of self-narration. "We tell stories about ourselves every day," Eakin writes. "Sometimes we can get other people to listen to them, but even when we can't . . .[,] this process of self-narration is constantly unfolding in our heads."[1] In quiet times, this inner monologue may be idiosyncratic and provisional, but Eakin argues it serves

DOI: 10.4324/9781003735595-6

useful, even "homeostatic" functions: helping us manage difficult past experiences, grounding the self in the present, and preparing for possible futures.[2]

"Jolting events"—like the COVID-19 pandemic—disrupt this process, sometimes violently, pushing private inner narratives into public view. Personal stories shared online during lockdown helped humanize tragedy even as they faced risks of exposure, misunderstanding, or erasure. Understanding these social roles of self-narrative is essential to interpreting diaries, as Eakin reminds us.[3]

By early 2020, Chinese mainstream media spotlighted personal accounts from Wuhan—the site of the first lockdown—highlighting grief, solidarity, and medical heroism. Yet the pandemic's proliferation of life writing invites a larger question: Do these texts mark a shift in self-narrative, or merely the increased visibility of stories that adhere to prevailing conventions? Given the dominance of biographical work, tight public discourse regulation, and narrow self-writing circulation routes in China, COVID-era autobiographical accounts emerge within a highly structured and deeply ambivalent context. On one hand, these texts suggest heightened interest in first-person testimony; on the other, they reinforce norms of service and collective sacrifice, mirroring pandemic-era moral imperatives.

This complexity is clear in pandemic diaries. While life writing scholarship recognizes that diaries differ from autobiographies, they remain key modes of autobiographical living—external traces of the everyday internal dialogue constituting selfhood. Diaries, written in real time, reflect daily fluctuations, shifting emotions, and limited information. In crisis, they become more provisional, capturing rumor, fear, speculation, and hope. As Brian Schiff calls them, they are "ante-narratives"—imperfect, fragmentary records preceding retrospective meaning-making.[4] Unlike structured autobiographies, diaries respond to immediate pressures: the need to record, process, and endure. Pandemic diaries become patchworks of speculation, rumor, observation, and emotion—some clarified later, others unresolved.

What emerges through this daily self-writing is not a unified narrative but the uneven, improvised work of meaning-making. Diaries do not simply reflect identity—they document its ongoing negotiation, especially under duress. As Eakin notes, this labor of self-narration matters not only for individual coherence but also for how we remember and make sense of shared history. In China, where autobiographical writing has often been marginalized in favor of sanctioned or collective storytelling modes, pandemic diaries trace a shift. They extend life writing's functions, adapting to crisis demands, documentation urgency, and political-social limits.

In the following pages, I examine the "autobiographical living" of Chinese writers—starting with Fang Fang's widely read *Wuhan Diary* (2021) and turning to three lesser-known voices: feminist activist Guo Jing, poet Ruo Shuiyin, and migrant poet Ni Zhou. I argue their social media life writing practices do more than chronicle pandemic trauma and uncertainty: they offer intimate glimpses of selfhood under pressure—efforts to steady identity, mark survival, and assert presence amid rupture. Like the *New York Times*' "Portraits of Grief" after 9/11, these writings transform personal testimony into public memory.[5] What is at stake is whether this life writing unsettles long-standing Chinese norms of self-representation—and I believe it does. Even under constraint, these voices of autobiographical living open space for once-silenced stories, redrawing autobiographical legitimacy and underscoring the precarious, vital act of narrating the self in crisis.

Revisiting Fang Fang's *Wuhan Diary*

To provide context for these diaries, I begin with bestselling Chinese novelist Fang Fang, who became an unexpected chronicler of the early pandemic by posting a diary online during Wuhan's 76-day lockdown. Her 60 entries, written between January and March 2020, gained rapid online readership and were later published in print publications and translation.[6] Rushed into global circulation with minimal editing, the diary was met with both acclaim and controversy—its rawness a mark of its original digital origins.[7] *Wuhan Diary* was not a solitary production but a participatory text, shaped in real time by its readers, as Gammel and Wang observe.[8] Fang Fang responded frequently to both support and criticism, transforming the diary into a public forum. Fang Fang included messages from friends, colleagues, and neighbors, creating a mosaic of voices, as translator Michael Berry notes.[9] This, in turn, constitutes "communicative and affective labor"[10]—a personal platform used to question structural failure during the crisis, as communication scholar Chen Chen describes.

What draws me to *Wuhan Diary* is its tension between private reflection and public expression. Fang Fang moves fluidly between anecdote and collective grief—sharing medical updates, tributes to frontline workers, and mental states. She is often reflective, even confessional ("Today I am actually feeling quite bad, and I think I really need to get some things off my chest"[11]), but the diary's most striking moments come through her rhetorical questions—unresolved, unanswerable, and inviting of response amid shared uncertainty. They remind us that autobiographical writing sometimes asks only that we sit with the unknown.

Throughout the diary, Fang Fang emphasizes the provisionality of her knowledge. She revises earlier speculations about the virus, credits reliable sources, and often apologizes for her language. Her tone is direct but rarely authoritative. This openness—what might be called a "diaristic vulnerability"—is central to the diary's impact. She does not claim expertise or moral superiority. Instead, she documents the struggle to make sense of events as they unfold—the core work of autobiographical living.

She positions herself as both witness and intermediary: someone with access and responsibility, but not above the crisis. She praises frontline workers and everyday kindness and condemns disinformation, official silence, and inequality. Though Western media often cast her as a dissident, the diary reads more as a reflection on the delicate balance between truth-telling and survival, both personal and political. Seen from 2025, *Wuhan Diary* offers more than a record of events; it reveals the complexity of writing under constraint: a writer negotiating censorship, scrutiny, fatigue, and ethical responsibility. Even under restriction, life writing creates space—for witnessing, questioning, and speaking from within crisis.

What is less known is that Fang Fang was not alone. Other diarists in China—some experienced, many not—wrote under tighter constraints, driven more by urgency than reflection. Unlike *Wuhan Diary*, these entries rarely imagined a lasting audience. Many appeared anonymously or disappeared with deleted accounts. To counter this loss, volunteers began archiving posts on platforms like GitHub, contributing to a fragile collective memory project.

These efforts highlight the unequal access to preservation, and how much depended on others to prevent erasure. Yang Guobin's *The Wuhan Lockdown* (2022), the most comprehensive study of this writing, profiles diaries from students, delivery workers, teachers, and COVID patients. He calls their work "endurance art"—less critique than testimony.[12] Their writing records fear, fatigue, and the fragile rhythms of getting by. This archive includes voices like Guo Jing, Ruo Shuiyin, and Ni Zhou—life writers who didn't seek national attention, but whose spare words capture what it meant to be sick, alone, and surviving in a city unraveling.

Guo Jing's Feminist Archive of Survival

After reading Fang Fang's *Wuhan Diary* several times, I've become attuned to its tone—candid, literary, restrained—and to the moral authority it carries as a document of public conscience. Yet far fewer people, even within my field, are familiar with Guo Jing's *Wuhan Lockdown Diary*, first published in March 2020 in Chinese by Taipei-based Linking Publishing (聯經出版), the first literary press to officially release a Wuhan lockdown diary (Figure 4.1). Despite its striking immediacy and quiet radicalism, it remains largely overlooked. Whereas Fang Fang's work reads like a civic chronicle, appealing to moral reason and public accountability, Guo Jing writes from a more precarious positionality: as a feminist activist, her entries often center interpersonal care, grassroots solidarity, and the psychic toll of structural violence. The "quiet radicalism" stems from not only what she writes but also how the fragmentary, affectively charged entries resist closure and invite lateral forms of empathy and attention. Bringing both diaries into dialogue complicates dominant narratives of the pandemic. It raises questions about authorship, visibility, gendered labor, and what counts as legitimate testimony in a moment of crisis.

One entry, dated 26 January 2020, stands out to me in particular. "On the first day," she writes, "I could not upload my writing and pictures to the Weibo account. I converted the text to an image format and managed to upload them online. Yesterday, I could not even publish them in my WeChat updates."[13] The entry goes on to measure the shrinking reach of her posts—5,000 shares one day, only 45 the next—and the creeping self-doubt that accompanies algorithmic silencing: "For a short while I thought no one liked my writing." That kind of vulnerability is rare,

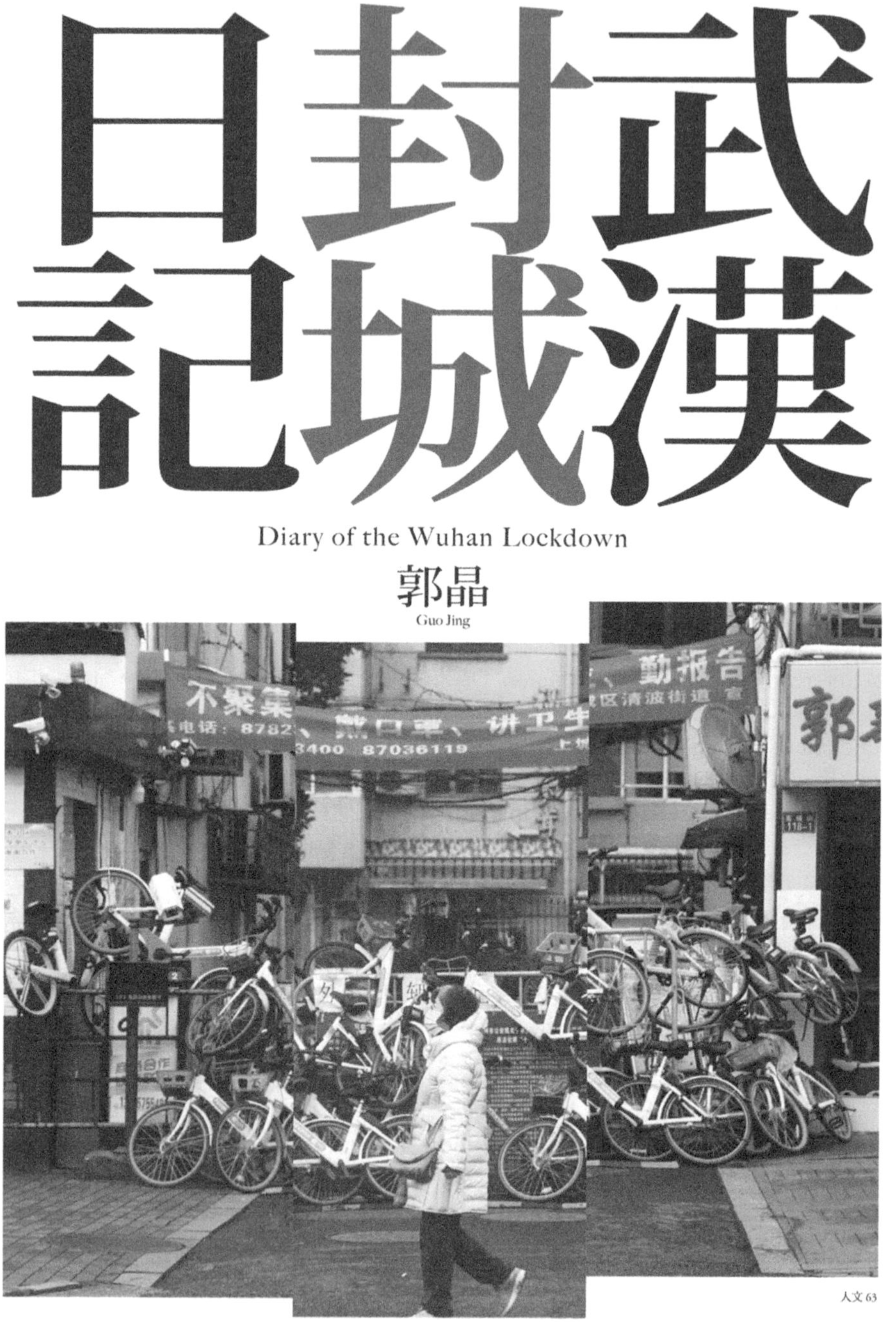

FIGURE 4.1 Guo Jing. 武漢封城日記 (*Diary of the Wuhan Lockdown*). Taipei: Linking Publishing, 2020.

and so is her technological savvy: converting text to image to evade censorship is itself a form of resistance. The diary is not just about documenting the lockdown—it *enacts* it, registering in form and content the struggle to remain visible.

The title, *Wuhan Lockdown Diary*, echoes Fang Fang's while expanding the archive to include a different kind of voice: younger, feminist, deeply attentive to the gendered textures of care, labor, and everyday movement. A widely circulated cover image (Figure 4.1) reflects this: a woman in a white parka and black mask walks past a locked tangle of bicycles, framed by commercial banners in Chinese and English. The stillness—the sense of being frozen in place—echoes the diary's themes of restriction and constraint. Her feet, in motion, stand out: the only visible sign of movement, they ostensibly mark the small, necessary actions that shape each day—like walking, like writing.

And yet—despite the clarity, intelligence, and emotional depth of Guo Jing's writing—it has received far less attention than Fang Fang's. Why? I often return to this question with unease. Is it the lack of official literary status? The faster, more fragmented style of online writing? The overt feminism, or perhaps the grassroots tone that doesn't lend itself as easily to mainstream publishing circuits? Possibly all of the above. But if we're attentive to what archives leave out—and who gets heard in moments of collective crisis—then Guo Jing's diary deserves not only to be read but also to be taught, translated, and remembered. It reminds us that history is also made from small, persistent acts of witnessing—typed, posted, deleted, and sometimes saved.

Ruo Shuiyin: The Weight of Responsibility

Ruo Shuiyin—pen name of Long Qiaoling—is a nurse from Gansu province in northwestern China, a member of the Gansu Provincial Writers Association, and a Communist Party member. When COVID-19 overwhelmed Wuhan, she volunteered to serve in a shelter hospital. Her poems, written under immense psychological strain, express something both intimate and politically dissonant: a longing to survive, not for glory, but simply to go home. In her poem, "Please Don't Disturb," she writes: "I just want to return home safe when the epidemic ends/even if all that remains are my bones."[14] "The slogans are yours," she charges in the same poem—quietly refusing the official language of collective resilience, and casting that narrative as someone else's: "yours," not hers. While state media celebrated frontline workers as heroes, Ruo's writing holds space for exhaustion, grief, and quiet desperation. Her poetry reveals what it means to serve while resisting conscription into a story you didn't choose. Though she did the work, she did not mythologize it. Her desire to return home—to exit the frame of sacrifice—enacts a kind of self-demobilization. She refused to translate her experience into the tropes of medical heroism.

In her haunting poem, "The Night of the Lantern Festival," translated by Ping Zhu and Chen Chen, a speaker sits behind a hotel window in Wuhan, breathing in the dark. The poem never explicitly describes the virus, the isolation, or the danger—but every line feels saturated with it:

> Room 8810, pitch-dark, a person is breathing
> Further and deeper behind the lights, there are
> more black windows
> as black as a cave, as the bats, as a gaping mouth
> as the lurking virus with a corona . . .[15]

It is a poem shaped by metaphor and atmosphere, written in the language of fear and watchfulness. The speaker's gaze turns outward across rivers and geographies—Yangtze, Han, Huangpu, Hexi—as if searching for something stable to hold on to. And then she looks upward, to heaven, "where celestials are feeding each other with long dippers." It's an eerie, almost mythic image, suspended between fantasy and faith. Finally, she dares to say:

> The darkness is still spreading
> Yet, I have faith
> When the moon of the Lantern Festival rises
> the world will be brightly lit.[16]

These lines balance on the edge of belief. It is not a triumphant ending, but it allows for the possibility of light. The poem, first published in *Poetry Journal*, has since appeared in collections including *Poetry Sky*, *Star Poetry*, and *Overseas Digest*. Ruo Shuiyin has won several literary awards, and her writings include a book of poems documenting the shelter hospital experience, published by the Writers Publishing House in Beijing.

Ruo's poem gives us a chance to discuss not just what autobiographical texts say, but how they say it. It reflects Eakin's notion of "living autobiographically"—the active, ongoing effort to make narrative sense of one's life. When that narrative is interrupted by crisis, the process becomes strained, provisional. In "The Night of the Lantern Festival," the repeated phrase "I look . . ." ("I look at the Yangtze River/. . ./I look up at the heaven") signals that effort to reorient the self through fragments of place, memory, and myth.[17] It's a searching gesture. The darkness spreads, but she insists on faith—however faint. As with so many pandemic testimonies, her poem leaves us with more atmosphere than certainty. But maybe that's the point. It invites readers to engage with feeling, to attend to gaps, to dwell in what cannot—or should not—be resolved.

Ni Zhou: The Precarity of Migrant Lives

My final example is Ni Zhou, a migrant construction worker and poet from rural Hunan province—about 300 kilometers south of Wuhan—who works in Changsha,

Hunan's capital city. His reflections remain anchored in the lived conditions of urban precarity as he critiques the instability and invisibility of migrant lives in China's rapidly modernizing cities. Contrasting the imagined safety of his "remote and backward" mountain village with the supposed sophistication of urban life, Ni exposes how development narratives overlook those who build the city but never truly belong to it. Unlike Fang Fang, who was financially secure and had access to reliable medical information, Ni typically lived on low wages in overcrowded dormitories, relied on word-of-mouth news among friends, and—crucially—had little access to medical care in the cities where they labored. For Ni, humor and irony became ways to cope with deeper structural vulnerabilities. In this, Ni's poetic voice—understated and autobiographical—is a hallmark of Chinese worker poetry—ultimately, speaking from and for collective experiences.

In his poem "Disinfestation," he writes about the corrosive effects of the pandemic, critiquing the paranoia and overreaction during the early days of the COVID-19 pandemic. Through the repeated and disorienting image of "disinfecting" trees, plants, houses, and even the air, the poem highlights a kind of excessive, theatrical sanitation that far exceeds actual need.

The poem culminates into these critical lines:

> truth be told, no one has been infected in our village
> but because on cell phones and TV
> All the talk is only about coronavirus
> it seems like the virus were already here
> in the village[18]

The line "truth be told, no one has been infected/in our village" underscores the disconnect between local reality and the media-fueled sense of crisis. Despite the absence of the virus, the constant barrage of news and phone updates creates a psychological pressure so strong that it feels overpowering even before the virus has arrived. In this way, the poem critiques how fear can become more invasive than the virus itself, altering perception, behavior, and the emotional climate of a place.

Likewise, his poem "Changsha, Today," centred on the city where he works in south-western China, uses the metropolis as a symbol of the profound changes brought by the COVID-19 pandemic. Once familiar and lively, Changsha now feels altered and unfamiliar, reflecting how the pandemic reshaped daily life everywhere, as the first-person speaker observes: "I find myself cautious towards all these things and people/I took no notice of before."[19] Becoming wary, he personalizes the global crisis, showing how even well-known places became strange and fragile. The poem captures the disruption, anxiety, and shared vulnerability experienced by the speaker and the city's inhabitants, making Changsha a powerful symbol of the broader human experience during the pandemic.

Unlike Fang Fang and Ruo Shuiyin, who were, albeit differently, writing from within more secure social classes, Ni wrote from outside—on the periphery of recognition, resources, and protection. His poetry resists the glorified narrative of urban resilience and instead lays bare the inequalities magnified by the pandemic. With subtle irony and sharp clarity, Ni Zhou's poetry becomes a fugitive record of classed suffering—a counterarchive of the pandemic from the perspective of China's most precarious urban subjects. Ultimately, his poems challenge the exalted resilience of city dwellers, revealing how the pandemic further exposed the social and economic inequalities embedded in modern China.

Implications: Life Writing as Self-Mobilization

To conclude, I want to return to the opening claim that life writing does not merely reflect identity but actively documents its ongoing negotiation—particularly in moments of crisis. As we have seen, the social media life writing practices of the autobiographical voices featured here go far beyond recording pandemic trauma. They reveal how selfhood is shaped under pressure—through efforts to stabilize identity, endure rupture, and assert presence in the face of uncertainty. In this sense, the alternate Wuhan self-narratives—no matter whether in diary or poetry form—broaden our understanding of pandemic experience and emergent identities beyond Fang Fang's widely publicized reflections. They foreground the everyday struggles of those who had little time to contemplate the grander political stakes of the crisis. In a world where public health became inseparable from state control, these writings offer a vital counterpoint—bearing witness to the realities of endurance, estrangement, and, ultimately, the search for meaning and assertion of new identity in a time of collective upheaval.

Multiple authors discuss how the pandemic highlighted inequalities in China and the resulting exhausted resilience. The juxtaposition of Guo Jing and Fang Fang raises important questions about literary status, values, and the politics of personal narrative. In the context of China's tightly controlled media, life writing—especially on platforms like Weibo during crises—becomes both deeply personal and inescapably political. The near-impossibility of accessing these diarists' stories within China highlights a stark divide: such narratives are often erased domestically while gaining visibility abroad through overseas publication. This dislocation complicates their interpretation and reception, as personal testimony becomes entangled with geopolitical meaning—even when the intent is primarily humanitarian.

A common thread among these writings is their negotiation of both the self and the pandemic—not as a triumphant overcoming but as an ongoing struggle with uncertainty. Many framed survival as a moral responsibility, closely tied to themes of selfhood. Acts of care—toward relatives, neighbors, and even strangers—became sources of meaning, forging provisional identities and communities amid rupture. Yet this narrative of resilience was often deeply ambivalent. COVID-19 patients felt depersonalized, reduced to QR codes and test results, stripped of autonomy over their bodies and movements. Public health measures enforced isolation while demanding public loyalty through tracking and surveillance. In this climate, the writers' and poets' personal storytelling became a form of self-mobilization—a means of asserting presence and identity in a system that sought to erase individual experience. For some, resilience meant enduring; for others, it meant resisting the demand to endure.

Yet amid these shifting identities, the imperative to self-mobilize—through care, resilience, and narration—did not always hold. At times, it gave way to self-demobilization: gestures of refusal, absurdity, or breakdown that exposed the limits of endurance. Sociologist Guo Shaohua noted the emergence of "moments of madness" on university campuses, where students walked cardboard pets or crawled in groups, dramatizing the effects of prolonged restrictions.[20] Such absurd performances exposed the deep fractures in the personal selves grappling with the pandemic and the social order. Similarly, the suffering of abandoned pets, left to starve as their owners were hospitalized, underscored the loss of even the most fundamental capacities for care. In these moments, the absurd and the tragic intertwined: "This is what we are reduced to," these actions seemed to say—yet they also reclaimed space for recognition.

To fully grasp the significance of autobiographical living and writing, however, we must also consider how these narratives circulate and endure—or don't. An important part of this study is what it means to think of these Wuhan lockdown diaries and poetic pandemic self- expressions as an archive—one that is far from fixed or complete. Many of these personal accounts were initially shared on social media platforms like Weibo, WeChat, and Douban—spaces inherently ephemeral, prone to censorship or deletion. Some writers later saw their works published in print or translated into other languages, giving their stories new life and audiences beyond China's borders. Others remain accessible only in fragments, or not at all, erased by time or state intervention. This patchwork availability challenges traditional archival assumptions of permanence and completeness. Instead, it calls for a more dynamic understanding of what an archive can be: a living constellation of traces, fragments, and contested narratives that resist full capture. The very gaps and silences in this archive reveal as much about the conditions of storytelling under lockdown as the words themselves. Recognizing this fractured archival reality is crucial for scholars and readers alike who seek to understand how memory, power, and survival intersect in pandemic China.

This archive also depends on a baseline of narrative and presentational control. Studies of Fang Fang's diary's overseas publication pull in two directions. Reader backlash forced publishers to replace editor-produced marketing with material from the author and translator. At the same time, that authorial control was undercut as critics in China sought to dominate the diary's interpretation. The escalating responses—from factual objections to death threats against Fang Fang and translator Michael Berry—highlight the risks of making personal stories public.[21] Consumed for their authenticity, such narratives were also scrutinized for perceived failures—whether the author behaved "properly" in lockdown, or upheld norms of evidence, self-presentation, and usefulness. Fang Fang's diary, its reception, and the performance of these norms unfolded in near real time for other lockdown diarists.

Personal narratives could be co-opted into official COVID accounts, used to promote policy and model public compliance. Paradoxically, self-narration—an attempt to assert agency amid constraints—also exposed writers to new forms of interpretive loss, as their stories were mined for meanings far beyond the ones that prompted them. Yet these alternate life writings show that even without Fang Fang's visibility, writers and poets used autobiographical living to resist the narrative terms imposed on them—evading, unsettling, and rewriting the norms of selfhood in a system that sought to speak for them.

Acknowledgment: I am grateful to Irene Gammel for her generous editorial suggestions, which significantly deepened this paper.

Notes

1 Paul John Eakin, *Living Autobiographically: How We Create Identity in Narrative* (Ithaca: Cornell University Press, 2011), 1.
2 Eakin, *Living Autobiographically*, 154–59.
3 Eakin, *Living Autobiographically*, 22, 32.
4 Brian Schiff, *A New Narrative for Psychology* (New York: Oxford University Press, 2017), 45.
5 Eakin, *Living Autobiographically*, 4–7.
6 See *Das Wuhan Tagebuch* (German, May 2020), *Wuhan Diary: Dispatches from a Quarantined City* (English, June 2020), and *Wuhan Nikki: Fūsaka 60-nichi no Tamashī no Kiroku* (Japanese, September 2020), which translates as *The Soul's Record of 60 Days Under Lockdown.*
7 Fang Fang, *Wuhan Diary: Dispatches from a Quarantined City* (London: HarperCollins, 2020); Michael Berry, "Afterword," in *Translation, Disinformation, and Wuhan Diary: Anatomy of a Transpacific Cyber Campaign* (London: Palgrave Macmillan, 2022).
8 Irene Gammel and Jason Wang, "'Why Has the Outbreak Turned so Deadly?' Diary from a Quarantined City," in *Creative Resilience and COVID-19*, ed. Irene Gammel and Jason Wang (London: Routledge, 2022), 27–38.
9 Berry, "Afterword," 361–62.
10 Chen Chen, "The Communicative and Affective Labor of Public Pandemic Diaries: The Case of Fang Fang's Wuhan Diary," *Journal of Rhetoric, Professional Communication, and Globalization* 11, no. 1 (2022): 5.
11 Gammel and Wang, "'Why Has the Outbreak Turned so Deadly?'," 32; Fang, *Wuhan Diary*, 82–83.
12 Yang Guobin, *The Wuhan Lockdown* (New York: Columbia University Press, 2022).
13 This and all diary quotations in this paragraph are drawn from Hongwei Bao's translation. See Hongwei Bao, "Diary Writing as Feminist Activism: Guo Jing's *Wuhan Lockdown Diary* (2020)," MCLC Resource Center Publication, April 2020, https://u.osu.edu/mclc/online-series/hongwei-bao/.
14 Ruo Shuiyin, "Please Don't Disturb," trans. Josh Rudolph, *China Digital Times*, February 21, 2020, https://chinadigitaltimes.net/2020/02/translation-poems-from-a-wuhan-nurse/?utm_source=chatgpt.com.
15 Ruo Shuiyin, "The Night of the Lantern Festival," trans. Ping Zhu, *Chinese Literature Today* 9, no. 2 (2020): 59–61.
16 Shuiyin Ruo, "The Night of the Lantern Festival," 59–61.
17 Shuiyin Ruo, "The Night of the Lantern Festival," 59–61.
18 Ni Zhou, "Disinfestation," trans. Pina Piccolo, in "'The World Has Grown Weaker,' Lockdown in the Chinese Countryside, Poems by Rao Jinhui and Ni Zhou," the Dreaming Machine, May 1, 2020, accessed May 17, 2025, https://www.thedreamingmachine.

com/the-world-has-grown-weaker-lockdown-in-the-chinese-countryside-poems-by-rao-jinhui-and-ni-zhou/.

19 Ni Zhou, "Changsha, Today," trans. Pina Piccolo, in " 'The World Has Grown Weaker,' Lockdown in the Chinese Countryside, Poems by Rao Jinhui and Ni Zhou," the Dreaming Machine, 2020, accessed May 17, 2025, https://www.thedreamingmachine.com/the-world-has-grown-weaker-lockdown-in-the-chinese-countryside-poems-by-rao-jinhui-and-ni-zhou/.

20 Guo Shaohua, "Moments of 'Madness': Cynicism in Times of COVID," *Global Storytelling: Journal of Digital and Moving Images* 3, no. 2 (2024): 39–66.

21 Michael Berry, *Translation, Disinformation, and Wuhan Diary: Anatomy of a Transpacific Cyber Campaign* (London: Palgrave Macmillan, 2022), 206.

Bibliography

Berry, Michael. *Translation, Disinformation, and Wuhan Diary: Anatomy of a Transpacific Cyber Campaign*. London: Palgrave Macmillan, 2022.

Chen, Chen. "The Communicative and Affective Labor of Public Pandemic Diaries: The Case of Fang Fang's *Wuhan Diary*." *Journal of Rhetoric, Professional Communication, and Globalization* 11, no. 1 (2022): 5.

Eakin, Paul John. *Living Autobiographically: How We Create Identity in Narrative*. Ithaca: Cornell University Press, 2011.

Fang, Fang. *Wuhan Diary: Dispatches from a Quarantined City*. London: HarperCollins, 2020.

Fang, Kecheng. " 'Rumor-Debunking' as a Propaganda and Censorship Strategy in China: The Case of the COVID-19 Outbreak." In *Disinformation in the Global South*, edited by Hermann Wassermann and Dani Madrid-Morales, 108–22. London: Wiley Blackwell, 2022.

Gammel, Irene, and Jason Wang. " 'Why Has the Outbreak Turned so Deadly?' Diary from a Quarantined City." In *Creative Resilience and COVID-19*, edited by Irene Gammel and Jason Wang, 27–38. London: Routledge, 2022.

Guo, Shaohua. "Moments of 'Madness': Cynicism in Times of COVID." *Global Storytelling: Journal of Digital and Moving Images* 3, no. 2 (2024): 39–66.

Han, Eileen Le. "GitHub as a Collaborative Curation Platform for Memory Projects of COVID-19 in China." *Information, Communication & Society* 26, no. 2 (2023): 340–55.

Picerni, Federico. " 'Poets, What Can We Do?' Pandemic Poetry in China's Mobilization Against COVID-19." *Asian Studies* 10, no. 1 (2022): 123–53.

Qi, Lintao. "Source Text Readers as Censors in the Digital Age: A Paratextual Examination of the English Translation of *Wuhan Diary*." *Perspectives* 31, no. 2 (2023): 282–96.

Shen, Chen. " 'Diaries in the Lockdown City': The Year in China." *Biography* 44, no. 1 (2021): 38–44.

" 'The World Has Grown Weaker,' Lockdown in the Chinese Countryside, Poems by Rao Jinhui and Ni Zhou," the Dreaming Machine. May 1, 2020, accessed May 17, 2025, https://www.thedreamingmachine.com/the-world-has-grown-weaker-lockdown-in-the-chinese-countryside-poems-byrao-jinhui-and-ni-zhou/.

Wu, Shangzhe. *Wuhan nühai Ah-Nian riji (Diary of the Wuhan Girl, Ah-Nian)*. Beijing: Lianhe chubanshe, 2020.

Yang, Guobin. *The Wuhan Lockdown*. New York: Columbia University Press, 2022.

Yu, Jinquan, Binghan Zheng, and Lu Shao. "Who Has the Final Say? English Translation of Online Lockdown Writing Wuhan Diary." *Perspectives* 31, no. 2 (2023): 297–312.

Zhou, Cheng, Haoxin Xiu, Yuqiu Wang, and Xinyao Yu. "Characterizing the Dissemination of Misinformation on Social Media in Health Emergencies: An Empirical Study Based on COVID-19." *Information Processing & Management* 58, no. 4 (2021): 102554.

PART II

Life Writing as Archival Testimonies

5

COVID-19 PANDEMIC DIARIES

Tracing Conditions of Appearance and Disappearance

Julie Rak

On 15 March 2020, just days before pandemic measures were implemented in Canada, I decided to keep a pandemic diary after reading that residents of Hubei, especially in Wuhan, recommended doing this to reduce stress during lockdown.[1] I also decided to track the progress of the virus in Canada, and so I recorded 304 cases and no deaths that day. Here is what I wrote, as I wondered about the future:

> We might all withdraw into ourselves, and will take up different pursuits. We might all rebel, and become tired of restrictions. We could become lonely, isolated. I don't know. That too will be something to see, what the virus does to us as a society—who we really are in the face of something like this, who we will be.[2]

Five years later, my early words about the pandemic seem prescient. The virus did change society and politics in profound ways. As I kept recording, I described what lockdown was like for me in my city, and I traced the steadily increasing cases and deaths in Canada until it was no longer possible to find those numbers. In the beginning, I thought that keeping a diary might be important if I did not survive the pandemic. Eventually, when the availability of vaccinations made me realize that I probably would not die of COVID-19, I continued keeping the diary to trace the social responses to the pandemic and figure out when it might be safe for me to stop social distancing.

I do not think that I was alone in what I did. The use of the diary form to track the pandemic's health and social impact was part of the response to a worldwide upheaval. Pandemic diaries not meant to be widely read probably were used to track those early changes through individual experiences of lockdowns, mask-wearing and sanitizing, doomscrolling, losing family and friends to the virus, online work

DOI: 10.4324/9781003735595-8

or no work at all, and vaccination (or the fear of it). Other people around the world probably kept diaries like mine to make sense of the enormous changes that the pandemic brought to almost everyone on earth and to stay calm in the face of those changes. But here my own story as a diarist ends, because it is necessarily obscure and is the story of a private diary that will not ever become public.

There are, however, diaries of the pandemic that are different from mine in that they were meant to be shared. Their conditions of appearance can tell us a story about two things: first, how diaries are understood (and sometimes misunderstood) as a genre participating in private and public spheres, and second, how the diary's close association with ephemera can send collected accounts out of the public sphere once they have served their purposes. Pandemic diaries collected for libraries and archives such as the *Pandemic Diaries Project* at California State University, the New York Public Library's *Pandemic Diaries* initiative or the Passager Books online *Pandemic Diaries* series represent attempts to collect and curate diaries that ask for public stories in ways that refer to and also push at the diary's own genre conventions and affordances. The social changes that the COVID-19 pandemic wrought within and around the circumstances of diary creation, collection, and circulation therefore have something to tell us about why, and how, diaries about a world event were made.

Before we begin to think about how the diary genre was used to for the purposes of pandemic narrative collection, we must ask: what *is* a diary? The answer is complex. In its simplest definition, the diary is merely a series of dated entries by its composer. But from there, things become more difficult. Desirée Henderson calls the work of diary definition a "research challenge" because there are so many ways to make a diary from dated entries.[3] Philippe Lejeune has pointed out that analyzing the diary genre poses a series of interpretive difficulties stemming from the nature of diary composition and circulation when diaries were not created in order to be collected.[4] Challenges for researchers include how to find examples of such diaries, how to deal with published diaries that are edited, and how to think about what happens to diaries once the occasion for making diaries comes to an end.

Most importantly for Lejeune, the rhetoric of the diary must be understood differently from that of other kinds of life writing because the content of diaries constitutes "a practice." The diary text is a "residue" of that practice.[5] By this, Lejeune means that the process of keeping a diary is not merely textual: the material of the diary is informed by life beyond the entries. In some cases, the elliptical rhetorical strategies within a diary are not meant for public consumption, because as Henderson points out, diaries occupy a grey zone between private writing and public writing, dependent on shifting ideas of privacy.[6] Diaries not written for publication therefore may contain rhetoric that is for the writer alone, a code that others were not meant to easily crack.[7] Many of the things that can be known about published life writing such as memoirs or biographies, including why they are made, how they are edited, why they end, or even if they are read at all, cannot reliably be known about diaries. Because their composition may not have been made for others initially, it is important to ask too what editing or even the act of curation does to the meaning of the original work. The afterlife of a diary composed from a historically specific situation can look very different from the circumstances of its composition. Because the author does not necessarily see what they are making as a readable text, Lejeune points out that "there is a gap between the reader's perception and the reality of what happened."[8]

When it becomes a text rather than a practice or a trace, a diary can be subject to pressures and expectations that can work to change its meaning. For example, the afterlife of a diary as a text can result in the idealization of the diarist as a witness, accompanied by an attempt to discredit a diary's authenticity, as was and is the case for Anne Frank's diary.[9] Or, the result can be an afterlife of silence, which is what happened in the wake of the 1918–1920 influenza pandemic, sometimes called "The Spanish Flu." That pandemic saw half the planet fall sick with influenza, and more than 50 million people died.[10] And yet, with the notable exception of Richard Collier, whose request in newspapers to send him accounts of the pandemic resulted in more than 1,700 responses,[11] it appears that few were eager to formally recall an event that affected every community in the world, and so there are no memorials to the pandemic in town squares and cenotaphs. This is probably why most personal accounts of the Spanish Flu, including those in the diaries that must have been kept, were not collected or published. And so, the lack of collection of diaries contributed to the forgetting of the pandemic, and of its documentation. In approaching how a "diary" in the pandemic comes to be, then, the conditions of its appearance include how it is converted from practice to text. As COVID-19 pandemic measures began to change lives, the impulse to collect "diaries" highlighted institutional expectations of the genre. Some libraries, intent on collecting personal stories about the pandemic, used "diary" to signal authenticity and the immediacy of eyewitness accounts as a strategy to attract contributors. The assumption was that diaries provided raw, authentic accounts of daily living, even though actual diaries were neither sought nor collected.

When a Diary Is Not a Diary: Coaxing and Collecting

In a review of politician Matthew Hancock's *Pandemic Diaries*, a volume about his role as the former Health Secretary of the United Kingdom, Gaby Hinsliff has this to say about the genre of the book:

> A diarist's job is to capture how it felt in the heat of the moment, however mortifying it might be to read in retrospect. Everything else is just publicity. Or in the case of Matt Hancock, who never actually kept a diary but hasn't let that stop him publishing one, a book concocted after the event (but before the public inquiry) with the help of journalist Isabel Oakeshott from a mishmash of old papers, notes and emoji-laden WhatsApps.[12]

It might say "diary" in the title, but as Hinsliff points out succinctly, *Pandemic Diaries* is a diary in name only. And so, why use that name for a set of recollections? Hinsliff's comments make sure to say why reading a published diary is valuable: a diary is meant to capture a moment without second-guessing or image management. A diary might be able to provide a sense of what it was like to be a decision-maker in a time of crisis. It could make its readers into witnesses. Because it is not a work of witness but tries to appear as if it were one, the labeling of *Pandemic Diaries* has the potential to mislead prospective readers who might be looking for an eyewitness account of the pandemic the crisis unfolds. As Hinsliff says, such accounts can be mortifying and even damaging to a political reputation. This is why Hancock brands the book a "pandemic diary" to allude to the affordances of the genre, but without the unfiltered quality that might engender questions about his leadership at the time. The book is really a memoir by a politician, compiled after the event, not during it, designed to put its subject in the best possible light.

Although Hancock's *Pandemic Diaries* is an extreme example of the appropriation of the diary genre, it is not unique. Online "pandemic diary" collection projects sometimes turn out not to be about diaries at all. For example, the New York City Public Library's "History Now: The Pandemic Diaries Project," begun in 2020 and closed in 2021, states as its aim the submission of what it calls "online diaries." But the rationale asked for oral recordings about the pandemic rather than diaries: "The Pandemic Diaries project invited you to submit, via an online form, audio recordings of yourself or your loved ones telling personal stories about life amid the pandemic."[13] The collection process began with the direct request to "Tell Us Your Pandemic Story":

> The pandemic has affected almost all aspects of our lives, and this project seeks as many unique stories as possible. We're looking for reflections on families and parenting, education and cultural institutions, business and work, essential workers, life in quarantine, #BlackLivesMatter and protests for racial justice, health care and hospitals, trauma and mourning, the recession, mutual aid, art and literature, community organizations, politics, and much more.[14]

The New York Public Library was in fact collecting first-person accounts of the pandemic in this request for stories, which amounted to "reflections," not diary entries. In a panel held on 15 March 2023, New York Public Library curator Julie Golia describes the decision to document personal stories during the pandemic happened because of what she calls "the polarized narrative" about the pandemic circulating in 2020 in the American mediascape, which differed from the personal experiences of library staff in their neighborhoods as they saw people get sick, die, and also help each other and support local businesses to keep them going in the period of lockdown.

Grolia says that requesting a variety of accounts about any subject and making that process relatively accessible would work against the stories of polarization.

She describes the process of story collection as one akin to fishing: the library staff wanted to "pull our net as widely as possible . . . and that's why we settled on the idea of catching stories" using a simple format to get people to submit their stories as oral recordings.[15] She calls some of the recordings the library received "elegies" that people made for loved ones who died from COVID-19. She then says that "we got poetry, we got music, we got anger, we got politics, we got parenting, and everything in between."[16] But what they did not appear to receive were diaries, or at least, Golia does not mention receiving any. The New York Public Library went fishing, in a sense, for any kind of recorded narrative (filmed accounts were not accepted). The bait they used was the idea of the diary, with its sense of immediacy and dailiness. But diaries themselves were not the fish that they were after.

The Cal State LA Library's Covid-19 Pandemic Diaries Project featured a similar imperative to collect "diaries" that were not in fact diaries. The request is as follows:

> The Cal State LA Pandemic Diaries Project, organized by the University Library Special Collections and Archives, aims to create an archive of digital diaries that captures the narratives and experiences of our campus community during the COVID-19 pandemic. We encourage members of our campus community to document their personal experiences and contribute their diaries to the University Archives. There is no better time than the present to capture your experiences.[17]

The emphasis is on documenting experiences, but these do not take the form of diary entries. In the "Pandemic Diaries Packet" contributors are encouraged to download, the format is that of a one-hour audio or video recording, with a transcript of what is called "your self-interview." A set of questions in the packet includes a prompt to provide the name and some biographical details of the person submitting the story, and a set of prompts about experiences during the pandemic, including the questions "how are you coping" and "have you had any revelations or realizations."[18] The format, therefore, is that of an oral history interview done by the participant themselves,[19] and not of a diary. Why call these kinds of materials diaries at all?

What the New York Public Library and the Cal State University Library teams were doing is an example of what Sidonie Smith and Julia Watson have called in the context of life writing "coaxing and coercion," where life stories must be produced in response either to a set of outright requests for a life story or, more indirectly, to ideologies and expectations that profoundly affect the nature of the response.[20] The coaxer or coercer might request a certain kind of life story. The storyteller has to respond to the request, and so they must tell the life story in the way that the coaxer wants it in order for the story to be heard, or in order to receive another type of benefit. Whether the context is a court room, where personal testimony must be true to be admissible, a bureaucratic requirement to tell a personal story of qualification and need in order to qualify for a government service, or a story of addiction and recovery told in a self-help group as part of the condition of group membership and the need to recover, coaxing and coercion create a set of social conditions for a life story. In extreme situations, such as an interrogation, the teller *must* respond with a story because of the threat of punishment. But even when the situation is less extreme, all coaxing has within it an important assumption: collecting stories always constitutes an ethical relation between the request and the response that works against any assumption that personal testimony is unmediated. The request always carries generic and rhetorical assumptions about what the story is, and how it should be told. But the notion that there is no mediation is, Smith and Watson observe, nonetheless widespread in the acts of request and collection.[21] Since the stereotype of the diary is that it is a work of immediate witness and is not for publication, the use of the term "diary" for other kinds of requested materials within the discourse of coaxing works to underscore the desire to collect unmediated personal testimony.

The Cal State Library and the New York Public Library participate in these assumptions about mediation and story collection. Both assert that they are collecting "diaries" because, as Henderson says, some of the most commonly held beliefs about diaries are that they are private, truthful, and unliterary.[22] These qualities are all connected to assumptions about what diaries are, whether these assumptions are accurate or not: that diaries are unmediated, that they contain an immediate response to daily events, and that they are confessional. Since the aim of each collection is to collect truthful, confessional accounts of the pandemic for historical purposes, the request for diaries rather than stories is meant to signal that fictional genres (which can include stories) are not requested. Although both requests say that any kind of personal stories can be collected, this is not entirely accurate because there are limits placed on the medium and type of story requested. The limits have a purpose: these personal stories are supposed to be true because they are imagined as part of an alternative history of the pandemic. The New York City Public Library request provides examples of what can be talked about in oral recordings, while the Cal State Library Pandemic Diary package contains prompts that are meant to direct the submitter to specific topics connected to the pandemic and its effects. The libraries are both after a specific type of data. And significantly, they couch their requests in gestures to the positive nature of sharing and confession as a benefit to the story makers. The use of "diary" as a term is meant to evoke privacy and the truth, in the context of that sharing.

These appeals, particularly in the digital age, are not unique to the pandemic and the urgency it imparted to institutions to collect stories. In *Story Revolutions*, Helga Lénárt-Cheng explores the increase in personal story collection facilitated by more access to digital tools and online platforms such as StoryShare and calls the aim of the calls to share online personal stories an example of "collective intimacy," a term connected to everything from the corporate use of personal stories to story collections made for the purposes of social justice. The purpose of collective intimacy is to engender feelings of belonging and collective action beyond one's own, immediate experience, because "collections of personal stories promise a unique way to achieve the double objective of collective intimacy, in that we can now mine large databases of personal experiences for collective insights while also creating a sense of belonging and intimacy."[23] The New York Public Library and Cal State Library are participating in this attempt to facilitate collective intimacy, with its twin goals of the preservation of data and the creation of belonging from the act of sharing data. The emphasis on "diaries" creates that feeling of sharing and intimacy necessary to facilitate that act of collection. Collective intimacy, ultimately, is presented as the benefit story sharers will receive if they contribute to the collections.

Once material was collected, were these stories shared, and if they were, how did sharing happen? The answers speak to the problem of collecting ephemera, defined by Anne Garner as the problem of definition (what is to be collected) and diffusion (each collection of ephemera will have different historiographic trajectories).[24] To this, we could add the problem of presenting materials once they are collected, particularly if the urgency for collection, created by an event such as the pandemic, subsides. The New York Public Library's Pandemic Diaries project stopped taking submissions 9 July 2021 and has on its site that "over the next several months, the Library will review, preserve, and process each submission. When that is complete, the Pandemic Diaries collection will be made accessible to the public."[25] But there is no further information provided on the site about when the diaries will be publicly available, or even how to access them. The collection does not appear in online catalogue searches. The panel about the pandemic, and its stories featuring curator Julie Golia, begins with the playing of an excerpt from one of the recordings, a heart-rending account by a man who lost his father to COVID-19 early in the pandemic. But that is the only submission one can hear without visiting the special collections itself. It is not possible to even see a summary of the collection, or a finding aid, online.

The Cal State Library Special Collections and Archives Pandemic Diaries project site emphasizes the importance of collecting and archiving material. Like the New York Public Library project, it also has no online examples of submissions on display or accessible through the library catalogue. But a student-curated online exhibit called "The 20/20 Experience" does include material by UCLA students from the Pandemic Diaries project, with this rationale: "By examining a selection of oral histories from Cal State LA's students, this exhibit hopes to highlight the personal struggles, community empowerment, and life stories of Cal State LA students as they navigate a world forever changed by COVID–19."[26] The exhibit includes a timeline of events and excerpts (written, photographed, and filmed) by UCLA students about different aspects of pandemic life, including the experience of online learning, economic hardship and social isolation, Black Lives Matter protests and student resilience. In a section called "remarks on remote learning," a video by graduate student Michelle Fanara describes the difficulty of tutoring visually impaired people over Zoom, accompanied by text also by Fanara about missing their "desk in the English department in the TA office" and missing working in a university cafe. The video has a text gloss from the curators about its content.[27] The exhibit is not focused on the Pandemic Diaries Project as a whole and is focused on student experiences, but it does allow for the video and text submissions to be viewed, listened to, and read. These submissions are described by the curators as "collective stories" that they share with a purpose: "We hope that by sharing our collective stories in this exhibit, Cal State LA can experience an important moment of healing, empowerment, and unity at a time when we feel distant from one another."[28] The aim of "The 20/20 Experience" is a high level of sharing to create collective intimacy as Lénárt-Cheng describes it, understood here as a call to belonging and to healing from the problems students experienced during the pandemic and during political protests that developed at that time. The stories are described as "oral histories" and as "collective stories" in a gesture to this intimacy.

Intimacy can only come, however, from sharing the materials. It is significant that the only public sharing from the Cal State pandemic diaries project is a student-curated exhibit. No other stories can be accessed because the initial goal was to collect for the future rather than to share in the present. As the appeal from Cal State to contribute to the project states, healing can come from sharing, but the goal of the project is to create material for future research rather than public access:

> Your digital diary will help us better understand how we as individuals and a collective community are experiencing the ongoing crisis. These materials will be preserved in the University Archives, providing future researchers with first-hand accounts of this historic event. Recording and sharing your story can prove to be a source of healing, empowerment, and solidarity.[29]

The diary form is appealed to by Special Collections as a work for history and research. Collective intimacy is stated to come from the act of sharing material in an archive, rather than the student exhibit's stated goal of sharing publicly. In both projects, the work of collecting is reframed as sharing, and the genre of the diary is reframed as a genre of public witness. The result is a relatively muted account of life stories, couched in the rhetoric of coaxing.

Assumptions about what a diary is are the "bait" to catch life stories and collect them. The positioning of ephemera as the accidental saving of material means, as Garner says, that it is up to scholars of ephemera to "offer input on issues of accessibility and visibility will be essential going forward,"[30] which means that currently, access and visibility are problems for collections in this area. It is easy for what is collected to disappear, or never be collected at all, by institutions.

Non-Institutional Collecting: Passager Books' "The Pandemic Diaries"

Passager Books, an American publisher dedicated to publishing the work of writers older than 50, represents a different way to create an online pandemic diary archive. The collection, called "The Pandemic Diaries," appeared in March 2020 as lockdowns in North America began. The editors put passages from writers' journals, photographs, and links into a scrolling web page. The format proved popular, with Passager reporting that their contributors sent in diary entries from many places in the world, so that "the Passager community became global, and each piece of correspondence added a new and important moment to the record."[31] There are more than 100 submissions posted on the web page from March 2020 to June 2022, arranged on the page in a continuous scroll. There is no index, and submissions are only roughly in date order. Passager Books does not appear to make many editorial interventions, except to format entries. Its submission guidelines, however, are very clear and include guidelines about word limit, a request for artwork, age limits for contributors and most importantly, they request journal entries only, and not fiction:

> Are you keeping a journal or diary during this pandemic? If so, we invite you to share an entry (or two) with Passager, a journal and press dedicated to writers over 50. We're interested in observations, impressions, feelings, conversations, encounters with people, and places, drawings, and artwork . . . please share an entry from your journal with us. No poems or essays, please. Journal entries only. Writers must be age 50 or older to submit.[32]

The tone is welcoming, but firm. There is an age limit, because of the focus of the press and its journal, as well as word limits and an artwork limit of two works only. The instructions go on to say when submissions will be posted, and how contributors will know that their journals are selected.

The resulting online collection has a range of subjects but all fall within the diary genre, whether the medium is visual or textual. Most submissions are called "journal entry" and are dated. Some record how many days in isolation. Some excerpts consist of multiple dated entries, while others are just a photograph or artwork with a caption. Since the focus of the Passager Books community is on older authors, who are among the people most vulnerable if they contract COVID-19, and on writers and writing whose words have been selected and curated, most entries are well written, are about specific situations and people, and often have to do with problems with aging and isolation during the pandemic. Topics range from the mundane to the profound, amusing, and even heartbreaking. For example, Rim Chon, from New York City, keeps an account of food and provides this excerpt:

> I've rediscovered cottage cheese. It's delicious and one big spoonful does the trick for a quick hunger fix. I've had baked potato as dinner more than I've had in the last decade. Instant ramen used to be a treat. Now it feels depressing.[33]

Debby Kaspari, of Oklahoma, provides images of paintings she makes of what she wishes she had, including types of food and a still life with rolls of toilet paper called "My Precious." Dorothy Rossi, from Colorado, muses on the doings of robins outside.

Unlike the curated collections in the New York City Public Library and Cal State, the Passager Books collection has stayed public and so has become a record of pandemic time from contributors in the United States and around the world. The public nature of the entries makes the site easy to find online, and so entries were international. Passager Books is a writer community, and so the entries are carefully written and succinctly observed. There is no way to find out how many times the site has been accessed, but it is relatively high in Google searches for "pandemic diaries" (placed before the New York Public Library project), and so it did have and could still have some readers. But how many, or what they think of the collection, remains unknown. The Passager collection therefore appears in an ephemeral half-light: its submissions record pandemic and lockdown experiences, but as the crisis passes, they may no longer be read at all.

Conclusion

Unlike silences and reluctance to collect personal stories which mark the legacy of the 1918–1920 pandemic, stories about COVID-19 were collected actively and, to some extent, remain legible and open to analysis. As Guy Beiner points out, this is partly due to the current interest in and technologies for public memorials: "Whereas the late modern era is marked by a growing obsession with public memorialisation, social and cultural remembrance of the so-called 'Spanish' Flu has been, by and large, muted and at times barely noticeable."[34] But the COVID- 19 pandemic does have some similarities to the silences that enveloped most accounts of the 1918–1920 events. The "Spanish Flu" was not remembered because there was no heroic narrative to be made from it. Why remember a pandemic that medicine at the time was utterly unable to stop?[35] The afterlife of those catastrophic losses has been one of collective shame, and so diaries and other accounts of the pandemic were rarely collected.

Our own era's growing obsession with public memory and use of online technologies created a different type of remembrance, which has much to do with the use of the term "diary." The advent of online video and textual storytelling has created the idea of a diary as a signal for collective intimacy. The term "diary" has been used to get some contributors to share their work. The labeling of online stories about COVID-19 as pandemic diaries shows us how the diary has come to symbolize a type of private witnessing in a public venue, straddling print and online registers. Therefore, it is imperative to think about pandemic diaries not just for their content, but to understand what "diary" means as a genre and how that genre has been used to collect stories, share them and sometimes, to allow them to become forgotten as the COVID-19 pandemic subsides.

Notes

1 Lily Kuo, "Write a Diary, Take Action: Hubei Residents on Fighting Coronavirus Anxiety," *The Guardian*, March 15, 2020.
2 Personal diary of the author.
3 Desirée Henderson, *How to Read a Diary: Critical Contexts and Interpretive Strategies for 21st Century Readers* (London and New York: Routledge, 2019), 7.
4 Philippe Lejeune, *On Diary*, ed. Jeremy D. Popkin and Julie Rak, trans. Katherine Durnin (Honolulu: University of Hawai'i Press, 2009), 31.
5 Philippe Lejeune, *On Autobiography*, ed. Paul John Eakin, trans. Katherine M. Leary (Minneapolis: University of Minnesota Press, 1989), 31.
6 Henderson, *How to Read a Diary*, 21.
7 Anna Jackson, *Diary Poetics: Form and Style in Writers' Diaries, 1915–1962* (Routledge, 2010), 10–11.
8 Lejeune, *On Diary*, 154.
9 Susan David Bernstein, "Promiscuous Reading: The Problem of Identification and Anne Frank's Diary," in *Witnessing the Disaster: Essays on Representation and the Holocaust*, ed. Michael Bernard-Donals and Richard Glezjer (Madison: University of Wisconsin Press, 2003), 141–61. See also David Barnouw, "Attacks on the Authenticity of the Diary," in *The Diary of Anne Frank: The Critical Edition*, ed. David Barneouw and Gerrold Van Der Stroom, trans. Arnold J. Pomerans and B.M. Mooyaart-Doubleday (New York: Doubleday, 1989), 84–101.
10 Guy Beiner, "The Great Flu Between Remembering and Forgetting," in *Pandemic Re-Awakenings: The Forgotten and Unforgotten "Spanish" Flu of 1918–1919*, ed. Guy Beiner (Oxford: Oxford University Press, 2022), 5.
11 Hannah Maudsley, "Remembering the 'Forgotten' Pandemic: Richard Collier's Collection of Personal Testimonies," in *Pandemic Re-Awakenings: The Forgotten and Unforgotten "Spanish" Flu of 1918–1919*, ed. Guy Beiner (New York: Oxford University Press, 2022), 53.
12 Gaby Hinsliff, "Pandemic Diaries by Matt Hancock Review—Rewriting History," *The Guardian*, December 13, 2022.
13 "Pandemic Diaries | The New York Public Library," August 1, 2024, https://www.nypl.org/digital-research/projects/pandemic-diaries.
14 The New York Public Library, "Tell Us Your Pandemic Story," The New York Public Library, January 22, 2025, https://www.nypl.org/research/resources/pandemic-diaries.
15 "Pandemic Diaries: Julie Golia, Julia Kwon, Jeremiah Moss, and Camilo José Vergara," The New York Public Library, August 1, 2024, https://www.nypl.org/events/programs/2023/03/15/pandemicdiaries.
16 "Pandemic Diaries: Julie Golia, Julia Kwon, Jeremiah Moss, and Camilo José Vergara."
17 "Pandemic Diaries Project | Cal State LA," August 1, 2024, https://www.calstatela.edu/specialcollections/pandemic-diaries-project.
18 "Pandemic Diaries Project | Cal State LA."
19 Steven High, Edward Little, and Thi Ry Duong, eds., *Remembering Mass Violence: Oral History, New Media, and Performance* (Toronto: University of Toronto Press, 2014), 5–6.
20 Sidonie Smith and Julia Watson, *Reading Autobiography Now: An Updated Guide for Interpreting Life Narratives*, 3rd ed. (Minneapolis, MN: University of Minnesota Press, 2024), 104.
21 Smith and Watson, *Reading Autobiography Now*, 107.
22 Henderson, *How to Read a Diary*, 1.
23 Helga Lénárt-Cheng, *Story Revolutions: Collective Narratives from the Enlightenment to the Digital Age, Cultural Frames, Framing Culture* (Charlottesville: University of Virginia Press, 2022), 22–23.

24 Anne Garner, "State of the Discipline: Throwaway History: Towards a Historiography of Ephemera," *Book History* 24, no. 1 (2021): 244–45.
25 "Pandemic Diaries | The New York Public Library."
26 Bryce Van Ross et al., "The 20/20 Experience: Impact of COVID-19 on the Cal State LA Campus Community California State University—Los Angeles," University of California State Los Angeles, January 27, 2025, https://calstatela-exhibits.libraryhost.com/exhibits/show/2020-experience/everychanging-uncertainty.
27 Bryce Van Ross et al., "Zoom University: Adapting to Virtual Education," University of California State Los Angeles, January 27, 2025, https://calstatela-exhibits.libraryhost.com/exhibits/show/2020-experience/zoom-university.
28 Van Ross et al., "The 20/20 Experience," 20.
29 "Pandemic Diaries Project | Cal State LA."
30 Garner, "State of the Discipline," 260.
31 "Pandemic Diaries—Passager Books," August 1, 2024, https://www.passagerbooks.com/pandemic-diaries/.
32 "Pandemic Diaries Submission Guidelines—Passager Books," January 29, 2025, https://www.passagerbooks.com/pandemic-diaries-guidelines/.
33 "Pandemic Diaries—Passager Books."
34 Beiner, "The Great Flu Between Remembering and Forgetting," 1.
35 Sandra Opdycke, *The Flu Epidemic of 1918: America's Experience in the Global Health Crisis* (New York: Routledge, 2014), 132; See also Beiner, "The Great Flu Between Remembering and Forgetting," 14.

Bibliography

Barneouw, David. "Attacks on the Authenticity of the Diary." In *The Diary of Anne Frank: The Critical Edition*, edited by David Barneouw and Gerrold Van Der Stroom, translated by Arnold J. Pomerans and B.M. Mooyaart-Doubleday, 84–101. New York: Doubleday, 1989.

Beiner, Guy. "The Great Flu Between Remembering and Forgetting." In *Pandemic Re-Awakenings: The Forgotten and Unforgotten "Spanish" Flu of 1918–1919*, edited by Guy Beiner, 1–48. Oxford: Oxford University Press, 2022.

Bernstein, Susan David. "Promiscuous Reading: The Problem of Identification and Anne Frank's Diary." In *Witnessing the Disaster: Essays on Representation and the Holocaust*, edited by Michael Bernard-Donals and Richard Glezjer, 141–61. Madison: University of Wisconsin Press, 2003.

Garner, Anne. "State of the Discipline: Throwaway History: Towards a Historiography of Ephemera." *Book History* 24, no. 1 (2021): 244–63.

Henderson, Desirée. *How to Read a Diary: Critical Contexts and Interpretive Strategies for 21st Century Readers*. London and New York: Routledge, 2019.

High, Steven, Edward Little, and Thi Ry Duong, eds. *Remembering Mass Violence: Oral History, New Media, and Performance*. Toronto: University of Toronto Press, 2014.

Hinsliff, Gaby. "Pandemic Diaries by Matt Hancock Review—Rewriting History." *The Guardian*, December 13, 2022. https://www.theguardian.com/books/2022/dec/13/pandemic-diaries-by-matt-hancock-review-rewriting-history.

Jackson, Anna. *Diary Poetics: Form and Style in Writers' Diaries, 1915–1962*. New York: Routledge, 2010.

Kuo, Lily. "Write a Diary, Take Action: Hubei Residents on Fighting Coronavirus Anxiety." *The Guardian*, March 15, 2020. https://www.theguardian.com/world/2020/mar/15/write-a-diary-take-action-hubei-residents-on-fighting-coronavirus-anxiety.

Lejeune, Philippe. *On Autobiography*. Edited by Paul John Eakin. Translated by Katherine M. Leary. Minneapolis: University of Minnesota Press, 1989.

Lejeune, Philippe. *On Diary*. Edited by Jeremy D. Popkin and Julie Rak. Translated by Katherine Durnin. Honolulu: University of Hawai'i Press, 2009.

Lénárt-Cheng, Helga. *Story Revolutions: Collective Narratives from the Enlightenment to the Digital Age. Cultural Frames, Framing Culture*. Charlottesville: University of Virginia Press, 2022.

Maudsley, Hannah. "Remembering the 'Forgotten' Pandemic: Richard Collier's Collection of Personal Testimonies." In *Pandemic Re-Awakenings: The Forgotten and Unforgotten "Spanish" Flu of 1918–1919*, edited by Guy Beiner, 51–62. Oxford: Oxford University Press, 2022.

The New York Public Library. "Pandemic Diaries: Julie Golia, Julia Kwon, Jeremiah Moss, and Camilo José Vergara." January 29, 2025. https://www.nypl.org/events/programs/2023/03/15/pandemicdiaries.

The New York Public Library. "Tell Us Your Pandemic Story." The New York Public Library, January 22, 2025. https://www.nypl.org/research/resources/pandemic-diaries.

Opdycke, Sandra. *The Flu Epidemic of 1918: America's Experience in the Global Health Crisis*. New York: Routledge, 2014.

"Pandemic Diaries | The New York Public Library." January 29, 2025. https://www.nypl.org/digital-research/projects/pandemic-diaries.

"Pandemic Diaries—Passager Books." January 29, 2025. https://www.passagerbooks.com/pandemic-diaries/.

"Pandemic Diaries Project | Cal State LA." January 29, 2025. https://www.calstatela.edu/specialcollections/pandemic-diaries-project.

"Pandemic Diaries Submission Guidelines—Passager Books." January 29, 2025. https://www.passagerbooks.com/pandemic-diaries-guidelines/.

Smith, Sidonie, and Julia Watson. *Reading Autobiography Now: An Updated Guide for Interpreting Life Narratives*, 3rd ed. Minneapolis, MN: University of Minnesota Press, 2024.

Van Ross, Bryce, Jocelyn Acostsa, Cyrene Cruz, and Keshy Jeong. "The 20/20 Experience: Impact of COVID-19 on the Cal State LA Campus Community California State University—Los Angeles." University of California State Los Angeles, January 27, 2025. https://calstatela-exhibits.libraryhost.com/exhibits/show/2020-experience/everychanging-uncertainty.

"Zoom University: Adapting to Virtual Education." University of California State Los Angeles, January 27, 2025. https://calstatela-exhibits.libraryhost.com/exhibits/show/2020-experience/zoom-university.

6

CROWDSOURCED

COVID-19, Life Writing, and Collective Memory in Latvia

Sanita Reinsone, Ilze Ļaksa-Timinska, Haralds Matulis and Elvīra Žvarte

In the centerfold of an unlined diary booklet, a pencil drawing (Figure 6.1) captures a quiet scene: a double bed rendered with steady precision. The headboard and footboard, composed of parallel bars, mirror the rhythmic planks of the wooden floor, all fronting the viewer—an open invitation into a private space. On the right side of the bed sits a young woman, thin-bodied and mohawked, dark eyes alert. She leans into a wall of pillows, her Apple laptop balanced on a tray beside a cup of coffee. A tall lamp arcs over a stack of books at her bedside.

Across the top of the opposite page, in bold handwriting: "Quarantine Day 14, Riga, Agenskalns/Baking omelets like a pro!" The date: March 25. A flurry of text in English fills the rest of the spread. This is a page from the COVID-19 diary of Anna Meiere Logina[1], one of many collected through the Latvian Pandemic Diary project launched just days after the World Health Organization declared COVID-19 a global pandemic on 11 March 2020. That moment marked the onset of an unprecedented global crisis. By June 2021, the virus had touched nearly 200 countries, with over 170 million confirmed cases and approximately 3.5 million deaths.[2] These staggering figures form the global backdrop for the local, human-scale work of our initiative.

Our project began on 17 March 2020, with an open call to the public to share personal reflections, drawings, and experiences of pandemic life. The Latvian Pandemic Diary Collection and accompanying PanDi text corpus were born out of this appeal.[3] Together, they form a rapid-response crowdsourcing archive of life writing, rooted in the conviction that a crisis of such magnitude demanded not only statistical tracking and policy analysis but also intimate, first-person testimony. As communication scholars Tracy Adams and Sara Kopelman have noted, the pandemic constituted "an unparalleled historical moment, one that requires an active effort to record and document the experiences of those going through it in the present."[4]

DOI: 10.4324/9781003735595-9

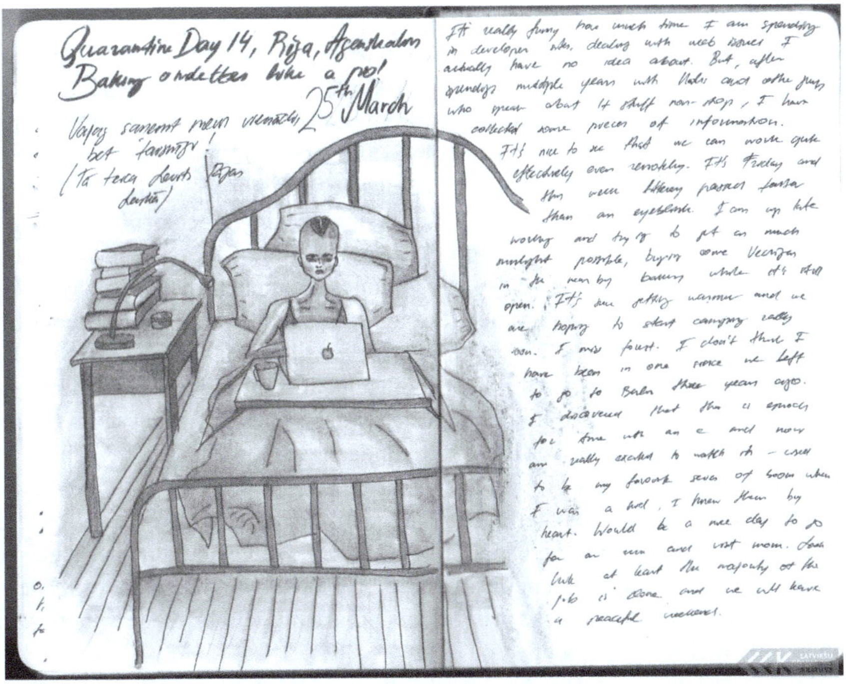

FIGURE 6.1 Excerpt from the Pandemic Diary of Anna Meiere Logina (ID 166–77), Latvian Pandemic Diary Collection.

From the start, it was clear that these diaries offered more than raw data. During times of upheaval—whether natural disaster or political crisis—life writing often becomes a mode of survival, a tool for navigating both the personal and the collective. In the context of COVID-19, we saw how diaries functioned in five key ways: as a means to structure daily chaos; to process emotions; to serve as eyewitness accounts; to create connection; and to preserve memory. In a world reshaped by digital technologies, such self-documentation took on new urgency. As face-to-face interactions disappeared, these forms of digital expression helped maintain a sense of social presence and community. The diaries became a way not only to record the moment but also to endure it. In the case of Anna, the diary clearly locates her in Riga's Āgenskalns district, known for its old-world architecture. Her scenes are domestic, even mundane—but in its quiet intimacy, it also bears witness to a time of extraordinary disruption.

This kind of entry helped clarify for us what the collection was really about: not simply documenting events as they happened, but capturing how people *felt* their way through them—how they responded, adapted, and made meaning in a moment of uncertainty. Throughout the process, our team returned often to these small, situated scenes—sometimes poetic, sometimes stark—that reminded us why we began collecting in the first place. This article argues that the Latvian Pandemic Diary project exemplifies how community-driven life writing, grounded in digital accessibility and archival care, transforms pandemic documentation from mere recordkeeping into an act of public memory-making—offering an intimate, participatory response to global crisis that challenges traditional archival paradigms and affirms the emotional, historical, and ethical significance of personal testimony.

Our team, based at the Institute of Literature, Folklore and Art of the University of Latvia, just outside Riga's Old Town, came together in the early days of the pandemic to respond to this moment through our shared expertise in life writing, digital heritage, and participatory archiving. From that collaboration grew the Latvian Pandemic Diary project. It reflects both a local response to a global crisis and a broader commitment to cultural heritage crowdsourcing—one that seeks not only to preserve personal narratives but also to understand how they shape, reflect, and carry us through moments of rupture.

Ordinarily, the work of gathering and safeguarding personal narratives—whether rooted in the past or unfolding in real time—is carried out by cultural heritage institutions, research centers, and public archives. As lockdowns swept across much of the world in March 2020, these institutions—museums, libraries, universities, and community archives—responded quickly.

Many launched new initiatives,[5] while others adapted existing digital platforms to invite the public to share everyday experiences of the unfolding pandemic. Supported by a growing toolkit of digital methods, these efforts sought to record not only the health crisis itself but also the myriad ways it reshaped daily life.

Looking back now, from the perspective of 2026, it is clear that the COVID-19 pandemic has been documented widely and in many forms—printed, physical, and digital. What distinguishes this moment, particularly from the perspective of museums, libraries, and archives (the traditional stewards of cultural memory), is not a lack of material, but an overwhelming abundance. Never before has a global crisis been so thoroughly recorded by so many people, in real time, and in so many formats, producing an overwhelming volume of information.[6] These participatory models align with what Canadian archivist Terry Cook once described as a shift in archival thinking: away from the idea of archivists as gatekeepers, and toward a more open, community-engaged practice. In this newer paradigm, archivists become facilitators—partners in a shared process of remembering and recordkeeping.[7] The Latvian Pandemic Diary project, which is our focus herein, was conceived in just this spirit: as a space for public memory-making, built from the ground up with contributions from those living through the crisis.

Other initiatives relied on more formal infrastructure—drawing on existing digital systems or embedding pandemic content into established archives. These platforms often enabled swift collection and public access, but their design sometimes limited the range of voices or types of materials they could accommodate. Even so, across contexts, there was widespread agreement on the urgency of documenting the pandemic. As ethics scholar Marc Kosciejew has noted, institutions such as libraries, archives, and museums bear a crucial responsibility to preserve the record of COVID-19—not simply for today, but for the future.[8] In his view, this responsibility is not optional or dependent on perfect tools; it is a moral obligation. He defines the attitude of these institutions toward pandemic documentation as a duty rather than a choice, leaving no room for hesitation or justification based on inadequate infrastructure. Most institutions that undertook such documentation recognized and emphasized the historical significance and potential uniqueness of this period in their calls for participation.[9]

As a result, the kinds of materials collected across these initiatives vary widely. Some projects focused on photographs, others on personal diaries, social media posts, or interviews. Many invited audio or video recordings,[10] written reflections, or even physical artifacts—homemade masks, vaccine cards, signs taped to front doors.[11] The most ambitious efforts like the "'Coronarchiv' Project" at the University of Hamburg gathered a mix of these, creating multi-format collections that now stand as rich, layered records of a time defined by uncertainty, adaptation, and collective endurance.[12]

Documentation projects can also be understood by how open they were—especially in terms of who was invited to contribute. As Chiara Zuanni has observed in her research on European COVID-19 initiatives, while many projects welcomed submissions from the general public, others were more focused from the outset, seeking stories from specific groups such as healthcare workers, schoolchildren, grocery store employees, or university students.[13] In North America, for instance (as discussed in chapter three of this volume), a number of efforts limited participation to residents of a particular city or region, while universities often concentrated on gathering reflections from within their own communities—students, faculty, and staff.[14]

Another important consideration is how accessible these collections are. In many cases, the materials gathered are stored in physical archives, accessible only through in-person visits. These projects were built with long-term preservation in mind—designed to safeguard a historical record for future researchers. But there were also initiatives that took a different approach, making collected materials available online soon after they were submitted, like the specially created platform by the University of Luxembourg.[15] These open-access projects were often motivated not just by archival goals, but by a desire to foster connection in real time—to help people feel part of something larger during an isolating and uncertain period.

The digital collections that emerged from these efforts vary widely. Some resemble virtual exhibitions, offering glimpses into personal experiences but with limited ways to explore the material more deeply. Others used more advanced platforms that allow users to filter, search, or sort through contributions—tools that greatly expand their value for both community engagement and academic research.[16] A handful of projects also released their datasets for public use, adding a layer of transparency and enabling further study.[17]

Just as the goals and accessibility of these projects varied, so too did the methods used to collect material. While a few still accepted handwritten submissions by post, most were conducted entirely online. Many relied on simple web forms or platforms like Google Forms; others invited contributions by email. Social media also played an important role—project hashtags, tags, and prompts created pathways for people to share their stories in ways that felt immediate, informal, and accessible.

Throughout this period, institutions around the world responded to the urgency of the pandemic with a wide range of documentation efforts—each shaped by its own resources, priorities, and sense of responsibility. These projects emerged at different scales and with different aims, yet all shared a common purpose: to gather traces of how people were living through an extraordinary time. The result is a rich and varied landscape of collections, marked as much by their differences as by their shared intent. While many focused on similar types of material, their methods and archival strategies diverged in meaningful ways. One project that stands out is the Latvian Pandemic Diary Collection. Built within an existing digital archive and focused on diary writing, it offers a compelling case of how quick action, thoughtful design, and attention to form can come together to create a collection that is not only accessible but also resonant. Looking more closely at this initiative helps us understand how documentation, when done with care, becomes more than recordkeeping—it becomes a way of honoring experience.

The Digital Archive of Latvian Folklore: Toward a Crowdsourcing Method

To create a model for rapid response cultural heritage crowdsourcing, this work builds on the Digital Archive of Latvian Folklore (ALF),[18] an open-access platform that has been expanding since 2014. Rooted in values of openness, participation, and public access,[19] the archive houses digitized materials from historical holdings of the Archives of Latvian Folklore—manuscripts, photographs, audio, and video recordings—alongside newer, born-digital collections. Everything connects in some way to Latvian cultural life, broadly defined.

The availability of this digital infrastructure was crucial when the pandemic hit. In moments of crisis—whether war or global health emergency—rapid-response collection strategies become essential, and digital tools often provide the only feasible way to gather and preserve testimony.[20] The Pandemic Diary Collection grew out of this necessity. It combined the urgency of a rapid-response model with the openness of a crowdsourced call, inviting people across Latvia to contribute to the "Diaries in the Time of Pandemic" project. The aim was to capture personal accounts as they unfolded—raw, unfinished, and in real time.

Crowdsourcing has long been seen as both promising and complex.[21] Even when the goal isn't massive participation, the process still demands care: clear communication, thoughtful engagement strategies, and a digital infrastructure capable of supporting participants along the way. Among the many possible formats, the diary stands out.[22] It's intimate, open ended, and well suited to capturing both the blur of daily life and the sharp edges of crisis.[23] Especially in the early months of COVID-19, when so much felt uncertain, diaries allowed people to register not just events but shifting emotions and evolving routines. As documents, they offer depth and variety—each entry a personal lens on a shared experience.

Several factors shaped our decision to focus the initiative on the diary format. First, we were building on familiar ground. The ALF Autobiography Collection—rooted in written life narratives—provided an existing methodological foundation we could adapt quickly. While we also accepted visual materials such as photographs, drawings, and scanned pages, at the time these were treated as supplementary because the platform and archival logic were oriented primarily toward text. Our aim was to build a coherent collection around extended, reflective self-narration, which diaries offered in a form already well supported by our digital infrastructure.

Second, the timing of the project was critical. We launched the call at the very beginning of the pandemic, when daily life was changing rapidly and unpredictably. Diaries, with their capacity to document lived experience in real time, offered an ideal form for capturing these shifts as they happened. We encouraged participants to write over an extended period to reflect the evolving nature of the crisis. This element of ongoing process was key to the project.

Third, we faced practical constraints. Although our digital infrastructure was solid, our storage and processing capacities for large files were limited. Formats like audio and video—which are increasingly common in personal documentation—raise challenges for long-term preservation and accessibility. Focusing on written texts, whether digital or paper-based, helped us manage the project sustainably while ensuring broad participation and ease of access. By keeping the focus on written submissions—whether digital or paper-based—the team could better manage and shape the collection.

One of the most distinctive aspects of the project was its speed. Diary entries were published to the digital archive garamantas.lv almost immediately—sometimes within hours.

Contributors could see their own words online and share them through social media, while others could follow diarists' experiences as they developed, almost like serialized storytelling. This created a feedback loop.[24] People read and responded. Some contributors referenced each other's entries, creating unexpected threads of dialogue across the collection. In a moment of isolation, these connections mattered.

Although we had prior experience with public crowdsourcing and a strong digital platform in place, this was our first attempt to gather contemporary experiences on this scale and under such urgent conditions. It was a leap into the unknown. Challenges surfaced quickly—from the difficulty of tracking scattered social media contributions to the strain placed on a small team already working at capacity. Still, the project moved forward, shaped as much by improvisation as by planning. In the next sections, we reflect on how we navigated these hurdles, what we learned in the process, and how the collection continues to evolve.

"Each of Us Within Our Own Four Walls": Designing a Collective Diary

On 17 March 2020—just a week after the pandemic was declared—we issued a public call via Latvian media, inviting citizens to document their experiences by writing diaries and submitting them to the Archives of Latvian Folklore's Autobiography Collection. Our initial announcement read:

> The aim of the Pandemic Diaries project is to explore and document through diaries how our society feels today—in a situation full of unknowns, where isolation is required and people are spending more time at home than ever before. However, above all, the goal of the project is to create a sense of community, reminding us that although each of us is within our own four walls, we are all in the same boat.[25]

Launched just as the first restrictions took effect in Latvia, the initiative landed at a moment when the virus—and life under lockdown—still felt strange, frightening, and newly documentable. Despite the already saturated media environment, the project quickly found traction. We appeared on national television and radio, and the call to participate circulated widely in online and print media. Other media outlets began launching diary projects of their own, inspired by the visibility and momentum of this one.[26] Much of the initiative's appeal, we believe, came from its tone: rather than emphasizing fear or catastrophe, we tried to foster mutual care and offer documentation as a hopeful, generative act.

We accepted diary submissions in multiple formats: emails with text and images; shared documents; social media posts using the hashtag #PandēmijasDienasgrāmata (PandemicDiary); and handwritten diaries sent by mail or uploaded as scans or photographs. Tagging our Autobiography Collection Facebook page or using the hashtag signaled a desire to participate, but we still followed up with each contributor individually to confirm their consent and discuss options for anonymity. Instead of limiting submissions to a standard form or interface, we deliberately opted for an open submission model, allowing contributors to write however—and through whichever medium—felt most natural. While this approach required sustained editorial effort, especially given the diversity of formats and the back-and-forth communication involved, it allowed people to write in their own voices, on their own terms.

From the beginning, we were transparent about the public nature of the archive: contributors knew that their writing would be made publicly accessible online and were invited to reflect on this as they documented. Diarists could choose to anonymize their entries or exclude identifying details—but most did not. Of the 238 diary authors who participated, 81% chose to publish under their real names, including Anna, whose story is introduced above.[27] Entries were released under a Creative Commons BY-SA 4.0 license, allowing others to share and adapt the content with attribution. This openness undoubtedly shaped what people chose to include—and exclude—in their diaries. But it also reflects a long-standing tension in the diary form. Historically, diaries have always sat somewhere between private and public, written for oneself but often with an imagined or actual audience in mind. Many nineteenth-century diarists, for instance, wrote with an eye toward posterity or circulation among family or friends.[28] The pandemic diaries, too, straddled that line: intimate, but also performative; self-reflective, but aware of being read.

Publishing diaries under real names brought a vital layer of authenticity and trust to the collection, as seen in the example of Anna's pandemic diary discussed at this essay's beginning. For Anna, and for many others, the diary became not just a space to record events, but a way of making sense of uncertainty—and of participating in something larger, even while physically alone. We felt this practice aligned closely with Philippe Lejeune's idea of the "autobiographical pact"—by signing their real names, contributors entered into a kind of agreement with readers, affirming their stories' honesty and historical significance.[29] As curators, we took this responsibility seriously. Together, we carefully reviewed submissions to ensure they met ethical and quality standards, steering clear of offensive or overly sensitive content. Sometimes, we worked directly with authors on small revisions, and in one case, an author chose to withdraw their diary entirely—a decision we fully respected. A few other entries were kept out of public view, by mutual agreement, due to their sensitive nature. Though not publicly accessible, these diaries remain part of the project and are preserved within our broader research framework.

Looking across the 238 diarists who contributed, we noticed a clear gender pattern: around 82% identified as women, 15% as men, and about 3% chose not to specify. This reflects wider trends in Latvia, where women often take a lead role in cultural initiatives.[30] While we didn't gather detailed demographic data, the diary content suggests that many contributors were Latvian-speaking, well educated, and culturally engaged—including creative professionals, university students, and young parents juggling remote work and childcare during lockdown. The diary format naturally attracted those comfortable with reflective writing, which may have limited diversity among participants. Our early collaboration with the cultural magazine *Punctum* likely also shaped the participant pool, drawing in contributors already connected to the arts and cultural sectors.

Over the course of 20 months, 238 diarists contributed a total of 2,333 entries along with 806 photographs and drawings. Most entries arrived via email—as plain text, Word documents, shared Google Docs, or scanned handwritten pages.

About a quarter came through social media, with some contributors encouraged by friends to share posts tagged with #PandēmijasDienasgrāmata on Facebook. This lively social media presence highlighted a core challenge for us as archivists: digital archiving can only capture part of a diary's life. Once shared online, an entry becomes part of a dynamic social ecosystem, much of which—comments, likes, embedded media—can't be fully preserved. In our archive, only the text and author-created images were stored; embedded YouTube videos, Spotify playlists, memes, or other content were inevitably lost. Likewise, reader responses—comments, emoticons, and reposts—often influenced what contributors wrote next, turning audiences into active co-creators of content.[31] What we archived, then, is just a snapshot, missing the fluid and interactive "social life" these posts had online. Capturing the full range of these interactions would have required technical capacities and consent processes beyond what was feasible at the time.

Importantly, this was not the work of our staff alone—it was truly a collaborative archival effort. At the initiative's height, social media users tagged the ALF Autobiography Collection in dozens of relevant posts each day. When we saw these tags, our editors reached out to authors to arrange inclusion in the collection, contingent on hashtag use. This flexible approach honored contributors' natural writing and sharing habits, fostering active engagement between authors and readers. But as participation grew, managing daily submissions became increasingly demanding. With only three full-time editors, the goal of making each diary publicly accessible in near-real time, complete with metadata and geotags, soon felt overwhelming. Though ambitious and well intentioned, this vision was unsustainable over the long term.

From First Wave to Fatigue: Patterns and Places in Latvian Pandemic Diaries

When we first introduced the Latvian Pandemic Diary initiative, we envisioned it as an open, ongoing project welcoming contributions for as long as people wished to share their experiences. Although submissions tapered off after the first year, we formally completed and archived the collection in an open-access repository by the end of 2021.

The busiest period came early—between mid- and late March 2020—during the pandemic's so-called first wave. This was a time of disruption and uncertainty, when everyone felt the urgency to document the rapidly unfolding situation. Many diarists captured the sudden upheaval of daily life: the shock of wearing masks, the experience of testing, and the anxious tracking of infection numbers. We also noticed how many found solace in nature, retreating to forests and the seaside—a response strikingly similar to patterns identified in Estonian diaries.[32] Parenting during this time stood out as a major theme, with many juggling remote learning alongside working from home.

By late May 2020, infection rates had dropped, and Latvia lifted most contact restrictions by June 9. Unsurprisingly, diary submissions tapered off. When the "second wave" hit in autumn, it brought a different energy—fatigue and a heavier emotional tone. We issued a second call for contributions, inviting both new and returning diarists.[33] While this resulted in a modest resurgence of entries after the quiet summer, the number of submissions was far lower, and the diaries' tone shifted—descriptions of illness, hospital stays, and losses replaced the early poetic reflections.

Looking at contributor patterns, we grouped diarists into three broad categories:

1. **First-wave contributors (82%/195 authors):**
   - Most submitted intensely early on, then stopped suddenly
2. **Dual-wave contributors (10%/23 authors):**
   - Paused writing over summer of 2020 but resumed in the second wave
3. **Second-wave-only contributors (8%/20 authors):**
   - Began writing during the second wave (October 2020 to April 2021)

This distribution really illustrates how diary writing served as a collective way to process crisis. The initial flood of entries reflected a shared need to make sense of a fast-changing world. But as the extraordinary became routine, that drive gradually faded.

Our team manually geotagged every diary entry,[34] generating 3,766 location tags across 818 unique spots. While the collection spans multiple continents, most references cluster in Latvia and Europe. Mapping these reveals more than just diarists' movements under travel restrictions—it opens a window onto their geographical imagination during the pandemic. Early entries often tracked global hotspots—first China, then Italy—and followed the ripple effects of border closures.

During lockdowns, many diarists turned to imagined geographies—dreaming of postponed trips and faraway places they longed for. Compared to other collections in the ALF Autobiography Archive, the pandemic diaries stand out for their rich geographic detail. Riga, in particular, is documented with striking precision—down to street corners, gates, and local road trips—making the collection feel like an unexpected pandemic-era city guide. These spatial narratives reveal the emotional weight of place and movement during a time when both were so disrupted. Through everyday walks and quiet moments in overlooked city corners, diarists shared how they adapted and found new ways to anchor themselves in an uncertain world.

The pandemic was challenging not just for individuals but also for institutions, including heritage organizations like ours. It quickly became clear that we needed new digital strategies—and that documenting such a massive social upheaval under strict restrictions demanded rapid innovation and flexibility. The Latvian Pandemic Diary project offers a valuable case study in this respect. At the same time, the collection's limitations—its relatively short timeframe and fairly homogenous group of contributors—highlight ongoing challenges in building truly broad and inclusive social archives. Even with national media promotion, barriers like unequal access to digital tools, limited free time, and the demands of reflective writing meant many voices remained unheard. These obstacles remind us that we must keep experimenting with more inclusive outreach and participation strategies if we want to create richer, more representative historical records.

Despite its limits, the significance of the Latvian Pandemic Diary Collection is clear.

What emerged is a layered historical record—rich with first-hand accounts of daily life, emotional coping, and shifting routines during a time of global uncertainty. As both personal testimony and cultural archive, the collection captures how people navigated disruption and made sense of changing norms. Its open digital format ensures these experiences remain accessible, inviting readers to encounter the pandemic through the eyes of others—one diary entry at a time.

Looking back, we remember not just the stories gathered but also the process of gathering them—the long calls, shared documents, and anxious coordination across screens. Our collaboration, shaped by lockdowns and uncertainty, was itself a way of coping. From those early conversations and the first perusal of personal texts—including Anna's in her Riga apartment—to the final upload to the repository, we worked to hold space for voices that might otherwise be lost. Ultimately, what we built together reveals the power of participatory archives to connect strangers, mark time, and preserve memory. But it also shows how much remains to be done. Future efforts must build on these foundations—seeking new ways to reach wider communities and to create records that reflect the full complexity of lived experience during crisis.

Acknowledgment: This essay builds on and reworks material first presented in Sanita Reinsone, Ilze Ļaksa-Timinska, Haralds Matulis, and Elvīra Žvarte, "*Archiving Uncertainty: Leveraging Crowdsourcing Methodology in Documenting Personal Experiences of COVID-19,*" *European Journal of Life Writing*, XIV, LD1–LD34. https://doi.org/10.21827/ejlw.14.42325. It is supported by the University of Latvia project "Open Knowledge Ecosystems for the Advancement of Citizen Science" (No. ZDA-LIP 2025/2). We are grateful to Irene Gammel for editorial input on this chapter.

Notes

1 "Anna Meiere Logina's Pandemic Diary," https://garamantas.lv/lv/unit/1418345/LFK-Ak-166-77.
2 "Number of COVID-19 Cases Reported to WHO," World Health Organization, archived January 19, 2025, https://web.archive.org/web/20250119183710/https://www.who.int/publications/m/item/weekly-epidemiological-update-on-covid-19-22-june-2021.
3 The digital collection "Diaries in the Time of Pandemic," https://garamantas.lv/en/collection/1415829/Diaries-in-the-time-of-Pandemic, while the PanDi text corpus can

be accessed through the CLARIN-LV repository, https://repository.clarin.lv/repository/xmlui/handle/20.500.12574/48.

4 Tracy Adams and Sara Kopelman, "Remembering COVID-19: Memory, Crisis, and Social Media," *Media, Culture & Society* 44, no. 2 (2022): 267.

5 Many European (especially Western European) initiatives have been brought together in a map. See "Museum Digital Initiatives During the Coronavirus Pandemic," University of Graz, accessed August 9, 2024, https://digitalmuseums.at.

6 Esyllt W. Jones et al., "Remembering Is a Form of Honouring: Preserving the COVID-19 Archival Record," *FACETS* 6 (2021): 550.

7 Terry Cook, "Evidence, Memory, Identity, and Community: Four Shifting Archival Paradigms," *Archival Science* 13 (2013): 114.

8 Marc Kosciejew, "Remembering COVID-19; or, a Duty to Document the Coronavirus Pandemic," *IFLA Journal* 48, no. 1 (2022): 20–32, https://doi.org/10.1177/03400352211023786.

9 In 1861, Lyman Draper of the Wisconsin Historical Society asked soldiers at Camp Randall to keep Civil War diaries—now among the Society's most valued holdings. The Society has likened its COVID-19 documentation efforts to this earlier initiative. See "COVID-19 Journal Project," Wisconsin Historical Society, archived August 9, 2024, https://web.archive.org/web/20240415232446/https://www.wisconsinhistory.org/records/Article/CS16333.

10 See "The Cal State LA Pandemic Diaries Project," Cal State LA Special Collections & Archives, archived August 13, 2024, https://web.archive.org/web/20231001144706/https://www.calstatela.edu/specialcollections/pandemic-diaries-project; "Pandemic Diaries Project," The New York Public Library, archived August 13, 2024, at https://web.archive.org/web/20240616060133/https://www.nypl.org/pandemic-diaries.

11 See "Czech National Museum Exhibits Masks Made During Pandemic," *Spectrum News*, May 28, 2020, archived August 13, 2024, https://web.archive.org/web/20240812220221/https://ny1.com/nyc/bronx/ap-top-news/2020/05/28/czech-national-museum-exhibits-masks-made-during-pandemic.

12 See " 'Coronarchiv' Project," University of Hamburg et al., archived August 13, 2024, https://web.archive.org/web/20240523211459/https://coronarchiv.blogs.uni-hamburg.de/?lang=en.

13 Chiara Zuanni, "Contemporary Collecting in a Pandemic: Challenges and Solutions for Documenting the COVID-19 Pandemic in Memory Organizations," *Heritage* 5, no. 4 (2022): 3620.

14 For example, at the University of Texas at Austin, students and staff could submit their information through the university's internal system and then it was published in a specially created website. See "Beyond2020. Living History," University of Texas at Austin, archived August 13, 2024, https://web.archive.org/web/20240520143256/https://www.2020livinghistory.com.

15 See "COVID-19 Memories," University of Luxembourg, archived August 13, 2024, https://web.archive.org/web/20240720123645/https://covidmemory.lu; materials submitted to the ETHOS Lab at the IT University of Copenhagen were published in a blog format—most likely after some review process—titled "Pandemic Diaries," ETHOS Lab at the IT University of Copenhagen, archived August 13, 2024, https://web.archive.org/web/20230206064053/https://ethos.itu.dk/pandemic-diaries.

16 For example, in the diary initiative of the State Library of New South Wales, entries can be filtered by keywords. See "The Diary Files," State Library of New South Wales, archived August 13, 2024, https://web.archive.org/web/20231009205447/https://dxlab.sl.nsw.gov.au/diary-files.

17 "A Year of COVID-19: Finnish Experiences of Everyday Life During the Pandemic 2021," Consortium of European Social Science Data Archives, Finnish Literature Society Archive, archived August 13, 2024, https://web.archive.org/web/20240812225002/

https://datacatalogue.cessda.eu/detail?q=3945864949e669e98a7586f743fa9cdfce591cdbbfc8519f5497b79eb421b978.

18 For more details on the Digital Archive of Latvian Folklore and its digital infrastructure, see Sandis Laime and Sanita Reinsone, "HUMMA.LV: Towards a Collaborative Digital Platform for Humanities and Arts in Latvia," *Baltic Journal of Modern Computing* 12, no. 4 (2024): 487–92.

19 Archives of Latvian Folklore has been a collaborative archive since its establishment in 1924 except for the Soviet occupation from 1941 to 1991.

20 See, for example, Sandro Debono, "Collecting Pandemic Phenomena: Reflections on Rapid Response Collecting and the Art Museum," *Collections* 17, no. 2 (2021): 179–85.

21 See, for instance, Mark Hedges and Stuart Dunn, *Academic Crowdsourcing in the Humanities* (Chandos Publishing, 2017); Sanita Reinsone, "Searching for Deeper Meanings in Cultural Heritage Crowdsourcing," in *A History of Participation in Museums and Archives*, ed. Per Hetland et al. (Routledge, 2020), 186–210.

22 See, for instance, Leena Kurvet-Käosaar and Maarja Hollo, " 'Is the World Still There?': Estonian Lockdown Diaries," *Biography* 44, no. 1 (2021): 53–59.

23 Anne Eriksen and Kyrre Kverndokk, "From Risk Semantics to Embodied Practice," in *Behind the Mask: Vernacular Culture in the Time of COVID*, ed. Diane E. Goldstein et al. (Utah University Press, 2023), 284.

24 It is important to note that the option to comment within the digital archive garamantas.lv is not enabled. Feedback is obtained when authors share their entries on Facebook or other social media platforms.

25 Our translation from Latvian.

26 For instance, the online theater magazine, "Kroders.lv" published pandemic diaries written by actors, directors, costume designers, and other theatre professionals, which were subsequently submitted to the ALF's Pandemic Diary Collection.

27 The decision to publish the pandemic records under the authors' real names was also largely influenced by the initiative's openness to archiving records originally posted on social media, where authors had already shared content under their own names, rendering the anonymization of the records largely redundant.

28 See Anne-Marie Millim, *The Victorian Diary: Authorship and Emotional Labour* (Routledge, 2013), 8; David Amigoni, *Life Writing and Victorian Culture* (Ashgate Publishing, 2006), 26; Rebecca Steinitz, *Time, Space, and Gender in the Nineteenth-Century British Diary* (Palgrave Macmillan, 2011), 2.

29 Philippe Lejeune, "The Autobiographical Pact," in *On Autobiography*, ed. Philippe Lejeune and Paul John Eakin (University of Minnesota Press, 1989), 3–30.

30 Jānis Daugavietis and Antra Leiškalne, "Self-Assessment of Cultural Literacy and Inequality in Society," in *Human Development Report: Mastery of Life and Information Literacy*, ed. Baiba Holma (ASPRI, 2017), 63–77; Sanita Reinsone et al., "Archiving Uncertainty: Leveraging Crowdsourcing Methodology in Documenting Personal Experiences of COVID-19," *European Journal of Life Writing* XIV (2025): 34, https://doi.org/10.21827/ejlw.14.42325.

31 Desiree Henderson, *How to Read a Diary: Critical Contexts and Interpretive Strategies for 21st-Century Readers* (Routledge, 2019), 141.

32 See Kurvet-Käosaar and Hollo, " 'Is the World Still There?'," 56.

33 "Pētnieki aicina turpināt iesūtīt pandēmijas dienasgrāmatas [Researchers Call for Continued Submission of Pandemic Diaries]," *Satori*, November 23, 2020, accessed August 13, 2024, https://satori.lv/article/petnieki-aicina-turpinat-iesutit-pandemijas-dienasgramatas.

34 The narrative map of the Latvian pandemic diaries can be explored in the digital archive garamantas.lv by selecting the "Places" tab. See "Diaries in the Time of Pandemic 2020–2021," Archives of Latvian Folklore, Institute of Literature, Folklore and Art of the University of Latvia, accessed May 23, 2025, https://garamantas.lv/en/collection/1415829/Diaries-in-the-time- of-Pandemic.

7

POSTCARDS FROM LOCKDOWN

Women's Pandemic Lives

Kristina Bhaun and Irene Gammel

"I completed my MSc in Computing! 😊" reads a postcard scrawled in purple and black ink proclaiming an unexpected triumph amid COVID-19's upheaval.[1] Another postcard, in stark contrast, presents a wordless story: a drawing of a female figure, her face a sad emoji, lying in bed—a bed that looms large in the composition.[2] These two artifacts encapsulate vastly different pandemic experiences—one of achievement, the other of illness. Both are part of a larger story, captured in an archive created from 2021 to 2022 by the Sheffield Feminist Archive to document women's lockdown realities.

Women—as primary caregivers, frontline workers, and essential staff—faced intensified pressures, persistent risks to their health, and greater mental health challenges, including anxiety and depression. This gendered inequity of the pandemic was of concern to the Sheffield Feminist Archive, a community archive launched in 2015 to document women's lives and activism in Sheffield, the largest city in northern England. Known as both the Steel City and Europe's green city, Sheffield's industrial past is tied to its strong community spirit and spaces, its parks, woodlands, and gardens. Reflecting this grassroots ethos, the archive is dedicated to preserving women's life stories and feminist liberation movements, notably through an oral history project that, by the time of writing this paper, had collected 50 interviews. But when COVID-19 hit, and public institutions like libraries and museums shuttered—along with the Sheffield City Archives, a key partner—how could women's pandemic realities be preserved? The answer was the Women in Lockdown project, which actively collected women's storytelling to ensure their struggles and resilience were not lost to history. A volunteer-led community initiative dedicated to "documenting grassroots feminism and women's lives and stories, past and present, in the Steel City,"[3] the archive responded to the urgency of

DOI: 10.4324/9781003735595-10

preserving women's experiences during COVID-19—particularly as many lacked the time to keep daily diaries.

The project's key initiative, Pandemic Postcards (2021–22), invited women to share their stories by filling out postcards titled "My Lockdown Looked Like . . ." and dropping them into blue post boxes placed in community and cultural spaces. This seemingly simple act—writing or drawing on a postcard—became a form of life writing. The period of collecting these responses coincided with a transitional phase of the COVID-19 pandemic, a phase best described as the mid to late stages of the pandemic. Lockdowns were beginning to ease, vaccinations were underway,[4] yet daily life remained unsettled—marked by shifting restrictions, lingering fears, and the uncertainty of what "normal" would look like.

Previous scholarship on the Sheffield Feminist Archive, notably by Lucy Brownson, Laura Gibbs, Jenny Kirton, and Sophie Whittle, emphasizes the archive's autonomous, volunteer-led strategies for documenting women's lives during COVID-19, highlighting participatory practices that preserved feminist heritage under pandemic constraints.[5] Our chapter takes a complementary approach, focusing specifically on the Pandemic Postcards as life writing artifacts. We analyze how their brevity, anonymity, and hybrid text-image forms capture women's emotional, domestic, and labor experiences, providing insight into the pandemic's gendered pressures. By centering content, materiality, and interpretive complexity, our study demonstrates how feminist archives mediate not only preservation but also the reshaping of lived experience and memory during crises.

To situate this analysis, it is useful to consider the postcard itself—its form, history, and communication function—which helps explain why the Pandemic Postcards were particularly suited for capturing pandemic experiences. After a full year of the pandemic, with embodied knowledge of its unpredictability, many of these postcards' creators reflected from a liminal space, both retrospective and forward-looking. They carried the weight of having survived a year of disruption, offering crystalized memoir-like reflections different from the immediate shock-driven, day-by-day diary responses typical for March 2020. As such, these postcards—created and curated for publication after a year of upheaval—assumed almost a commemorative function, marking not just survival but the transformation of the experience over time—a summing up of how daily life was reshaped and how the long-term impact of the pandemic started to be understood in personal, intimate terms. Today, the archive's 156 digitized postcards provide an invaluable record of how personal experiences intertwined with broader social, political, and economic forces.

The postcard itself suggests brevity—a distillation of thought, and a focus on essentials. Its limited space enforces conciseness, eliminating excessive elaboration. Unlike the letter format, it does not demand a lengthy composition, yet it still carries a sense of personal connection. Postcards emerged in the mid-nineteenth century, with Austria issuing the first official Correspondenz-Karte in 1869, which was a plain card with space for a short message. By the 1890s, illustrated postcards gained popularity, especially after the 1900 Paris Exposition.

Postcards are typically tied to tourism, with the recto depicting a destination and the verso carrying messages to loved ones—often reassuring them of the traveler's well-being. This practice extended to times of upheaval in the early twentieth century, as seen in the countless postcards from World War I, where soldiers and prisoners assured families of their survival. The postcard's brevity makes it suited for moments of crisis, offering reassurance, connection, and a tangible record of experience. This function persisted into the twenty-first century, as seen in the Sheffield women's project during the COVID-19 pandemic.

After a year of isolation, selecting, writing, and submitting a postcard to one of the specially provided community mailboxes required considerably more effort than a quick digital message, making it a deliberate, if brief, act of reflection. The format itself is unconventional and eye-catching, an open canvas for contributors to tell their distilled story. Though many participants chose to draw their responses, the postcards exhibit a raw, DIY aesthetic, with little evidence of professional design or skills. Indeed, the human hand is central—writing and drawing merge into a singular message to the addressee. These postcards lack the classic two- sidedness, their texts and images coexisting on the same surface.

Now, in 2025, the collected corpus stands as both a personal artifact and a historical record—revealing how women in Sheffield articulated their lives and struggles, documenting their realities, and built feminist communities through self-writing. Thus, this chapter examines Pandemic Postcards as part of a larger tradition of both self-writing and communicating during upheaval, illustrating Jacques Derrida's argument, in *The Post Card: From Socrates to Freud* (1980), which sees the postcard as a symbol of communication's inherent instability. Unlike a sealed letter, a postcard is exposed—it can be read by anyone who handles it. This openness disrupts and complicates the traditional sender-receiver model and reflects Derrida's broader critique of fixed meaning in language. For Derrida, the postcard also challenges the notion of a stable authorial voice. Always already out of the author's hands, the postcard resists control.[6]

Derrida's insights resonate with this archive: these postcards echo the crisis itself—inscribing loss of control, instability, and disrupted communication. But what, specifically, is the connection between these postcards and the feminist archive? To explore this, we bring together theories of life writing, COVID-19 studies, and feminist archival practices. By focusing on these inscriptions, we argue that these postcards do more than preserve history and memory—they create spaces for grief, community, and imagining more equitable futures. More than recount lived experience—they remake it, capturing the play of presence and absence, uncertainty and expression, in ways that define self-inscription itself. Yet, they also ultimately challenge the idea that life writing—whether textual or visual—can ever be fully transparent or complete.

Anonymous Voices: Pandemic Postcards as Life Writing

The method of collecting women's postcards was straightforward. In March 2021, the Sheffield Feminist Archive invited women to reflect on the impact of COVID-19 and express their individual experiences. Each postcard features preprinted text prompting participants to share their experiences:

MY LOCKDOWN LOOKED LIKE . . .
This postcard is a canvas! Write or draw something that represents life in lockdown for you.

At the bottom right corner, a pre-printed #WomenInLockdown hashtag marked each postcard, while the bottom left indicated that the postcards would be published in the Sheffield Feminist Archives via WordPress. The limited space of postcards mirrored the constrained time available to women during the pandemic, forcing them to condense complex experiences into brief, impactful representations. Postcards are sequentially organized in carousel 1 from #1 to #88, and in carousel 2 from 1 to # 68, the postcards remained anonymous—though at least one participant signed hers as "Fiona."[7] Unless explicitly stated, no dates provided insight into when they were created. As a result, these postcards lacked two defining features of traditional postcards: the sender's name and a timestamp, although they do feature the recipient's digital address on the recto. What remained, however, was the personal act of handwriting or drawing—a message crafted by an individual for a clearly identified addressee: the Sheffield Feminist Archive. By depositing these postcards into specially provided blue mailboxes available in community spaces—distinct from the regular red postal mailboxes in Britain, contributors submitted their lockdown lives postcards for digital publication, thus transforming private reflections into public records, joining a collective historical narrative.

Submitting an anonymous postcard differs significantly from diary or memoir writing, where authors typically claim their experiences by name. Diaries unfold organically, while the postcard's prompt—"My Lockdown Looked Like . . ."—imposes a rhetorical structure, framing the response as the completion of an unfinished task. In this way, the Sheffield Postcard Project echoes the directive-based collections of the New York Public Library and Cal State University Library teams, as discussed in Julie Rak's chapter. Unlike those initiatives, however, the Sheffield project does not solicit diaries. Instead, it aligns with what Sidonie Smith and Julia Watson call "coaxing and coercing" in life writing,[8] where the request for personal narratives shapes the response—its single-card constraint imposing both creative limits and expressive urgency.

Methodologically, a key feature of these pandemic postcards is their anonymity—most remain unsigned, despite revealing intimate details of personal and family life. This suggests that the women created them for *themselves*, knowing they would later be shared publicly. By doing so, they privately joined a feminist community dedicated to sharing—and proclaiming—their experiences during COVID-19. These postcards, as forms of self- presentation, resemble how people use avatars or selfies to project aspects of themselves. Yet by submitting their postcards to a feminist archive—an institution safeguarding historically significant materials—they also gave their experiences and sacrifices validation. Writing for themselves, they marked personal milestones, whether acknowledging a breakup or emphasizing the severity of the pandemic, ultimately using the postcard to protect what might otherwise be ephemeral, thereby acknowledging and commemorating their role in an historical event.

This combination of solicitation and anonymity recalls the Mass Observation Project during and after World War II, which sought to document everyday life, particularly among marginalized working-class communities. As James Hinton details in *The Mass Observers: A History 1937–49* (2013), the project's use of open-ended questions aimed to capture the routines of ordinary people during turbulent times—how they lived, worked, and entertained themselves? The archive's participatory model sought to create a democratic history "from below," allowing contributors to share authentic life stories without pressures of self-censorship,[9] a contrast to the less anonymous oral history projects. Anonymity, as Erving Goffman suggests, reduces the burden of "face work" in social interactions.[10] Similar dynamics are seen on social media platforms like Reddit,[11] where avatars and pseudonyms create an "identity playground,"[12] balancing personal agency with social expectations. The Sheffield women's postcards reflect some of these same principles.

So how do women use writing and drawing to tell their pandemic stories? How do they represent domestic life, civic engagement, or romantic relationships? What themes emerge across the 156 submissions? The postcards selected below reflect the rawness and spontaneity of untrained writers and draftswomen—artistic expressions that resemble Art Brut. The absence of a signature raises further questions. Does anonymity make participants more willing to submit their work? Does it offer them the freedom to express darker or more unsettling reflections on the pandemic—thoughts they might hesitate to share otherwise? In other words, does this project give voice to those who are neither "mainstream" nor cast as pandemic "heroes"?

The Archive of Women's Work: Domestic, Emotional, Artistic

The Sheffield Feminist Archive's collection of 156 COVID-19 postcards present a striking departure from tradition: each displays only the front—contrasting conventional postcards, which feature both recto and verso. Here, the recipient's address is prominently placed on the recto, framing each entry like a fixed point in an otherwise fluid exchange. Yet, the sender's signature is absent in all but one—a rare exception signed by Fiona. Only a single postcard bears a date: December 2021, a temporal marker of heartbreak, signaling the breakup of a relationship. This absence of names and dates heightens the archive's anonymity and collective voice.

Contributors expressed themselves in diverse ways: 63 relied solely on text, while another 63 blended writing with drawings, emojis, and other visual elements, crafting hybrid records of pandemic life. A notable 30 postcards—nearly a fifth—abandoned words entirely, speaking only through images. Even those who wrote often fragmented their thoughts, clustering words to emphasize key themes of the pandemic.

The postcards reveal how the pandemic reshaped everyday life, with communal themes of isolation, work, and mental health recurring throughout the archive. Isolation and loneliness surface not only as struggles but also as sites of dark humor, as seen in a quip about, "Becoming a/master of/masterbation/ 😊" (postcard #18). The weight of domestic life is tangible, appearing in 25 postcards, captured through the depiction of household objects and cluttered workspaces. Another 25 focused on the shifting landscape of work, illustrating crowded tables, home offices, and the ever-present glow of computer screens. Mental health found a voice in 16 postcards—about 10% of the archive—depicting anxiety (postcards #32 and #33) and depression (postcard #41, Figure 7.1). Yet, resilience and self-care thread through the collection, whether through mindful activities like knitting (postcard #53), video games, gardening (postcard #34), or simple walks outside. Quieter forms of coping surface too—TV, alcohol (postcard #43), and drug use (postcard #56).

Safety measures emerge as an omnipresent motif, with multiple postcards addressing mask-wearing (postcards #71 and #87). Loss is woven throughout: some speak of losing a job (postcard #44), others of losing loved ones—including the grief of a lost parent (postcard #75). The identity of Sheffield as a university town echoes throughout, as some postcards reflect both the upheaval of higher

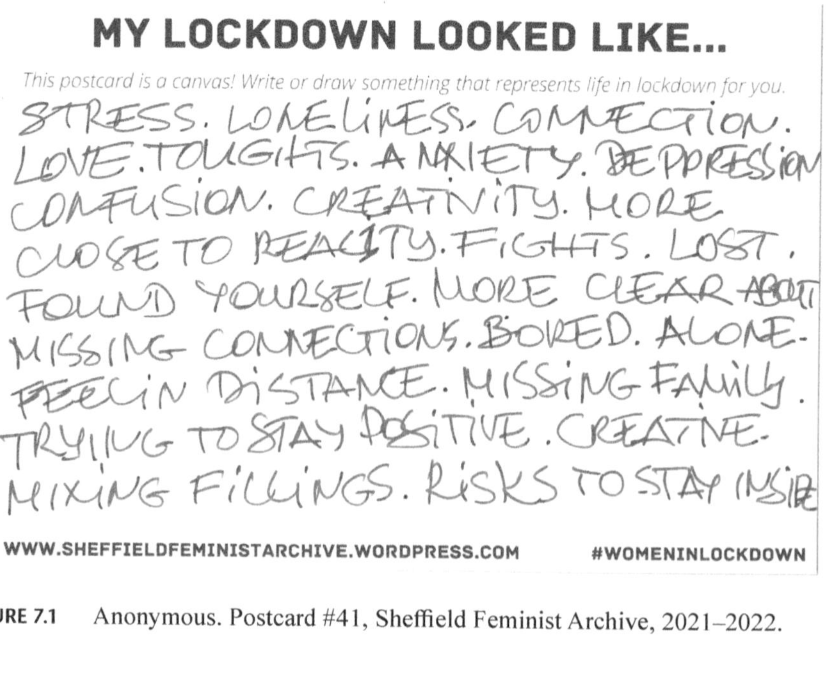

FIGURE 7.1 Anonymous. Postcard #41, Sheffield Feminist Archive, 2021–2022.

education and the pleasure of education (postcards #73 and #46). Digital technology appears prominently across the collection, its presence unrelenting in depictions of video calls (postcards #62 and #81, Figure 7.2), Zoom meetings, and the omnipresence of screens. Together, these cards offer distilled self-portraits of life under COVID-19. Since each postcard is intended to be archived and exhibited publicly, contributing one can be seen as a feminist act of self-assertion. Even in anonymity, creators ensure that distilled records of their pandemic lives become part of the historical archiving of women's lives during the pandemic.

Consider postcard #11 (Figure 7.3), a powerful visual self-representation of an anonymous woman navigating the demands of domesticity. She takes up the full postcard, depicted in profile with shoulder-length hair and wide-open eyes.[13] Surrounding her, five figures clamor for attention: an adult male figure and three toddlers, one with a bottle, each with open mouths. Arrows from each face converge upon her, embodying the relentless demands on her time and energy as a mother and wife, reinforcing Breanne Fahs's feminist COVID-19 study on women's doubled and tripled emotional, sexual, and domestic labour.[14] Yet, despite the visual cacophony, she remains silent, the only one not vocalizing—a blunt depiction of her emotional isolation. One arrow disturbingly doubles as a knife, underscoring the sharp toll of this labor and the political and ethical weight of drawn life writing, particularly in feminist and trauma narratives.[15] It reminds us that visual representation—especially drawing—can speak where language fails. In *Graphic Women: Life Narrative and Contemporary Comics* (2010), Hillary Chute argues that

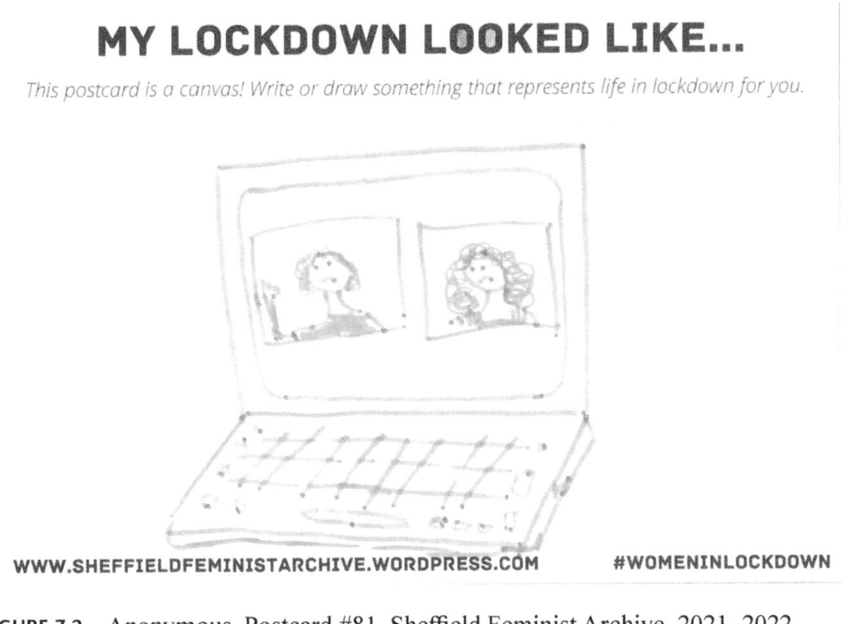

FIGURE 7.2 Anonymous. Postcard #81, Sheffield Feminist Archive, 2021–2022.

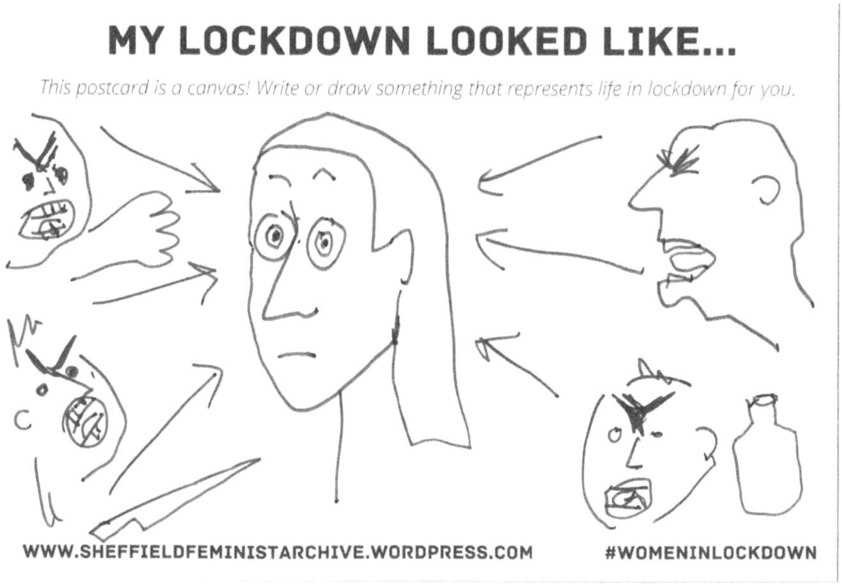

FIGURE 7.3 Anonymous. Postcard #11, Sheffield Feminist Archive, 2021–2022.

the materiality of drawing—with its visible inscription, erasures, and revisions—creates a layered, fragmented, and open-ended form of self-representation. Here, too, the drawing offers a spatialized approach to storytelling, revealing memory's unstable construction in ways prose alone cannot.

The pandemic lockdown exposed and intensified the invisible labor that women perform, particularly the emotional and relational labor required to sustain both households and professional lives. Postcard #26 (Figure 7.4) depicts an expressionless woman cradling a baby while working at a computer desk, her body overlaid with the handwritten words "TOUCHED OUT." A child yells "MUUUM!" in the background. Every inch of the card brims with demands, as handwritten words bombard the central figure: "lack of support, teaching at home, deadlines, exhaustion, no social life, money, claustrophobia, anxiety, breastfeeding while doing PhD research, overwhelmed."[16] In each postcard, relational labor dominates the imagery, and in each, the central female figure is both present and absent, her identity fractured by competing demands.

Postcard #7 (Figure 7.5) captures a young girl sitting at a large dinner table, her math homework open before her. One side of the workbook contains multiplication problems, and the other reads "work it out," a single tear rolling down her cheek.[17] The postcard viscerally conveys the shared strain of COVID-19 lockdowns: both mother and child are burdened, trapped in the upheaval of disrupted routines. This scene reinforces Kathryn Asbury and colleagues' observation that

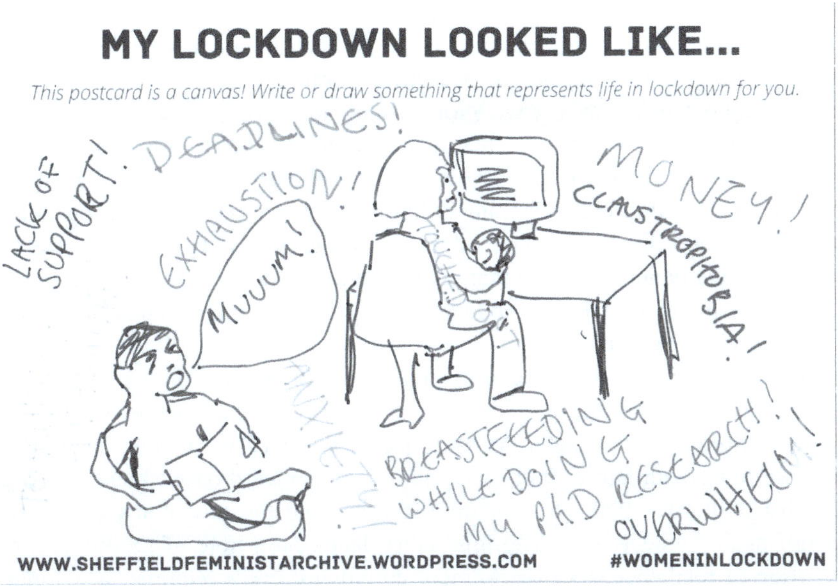

FIGURE 7.4 Anonymous. Postcard #26, Sheffield Feminist Archive, 2021–2022.

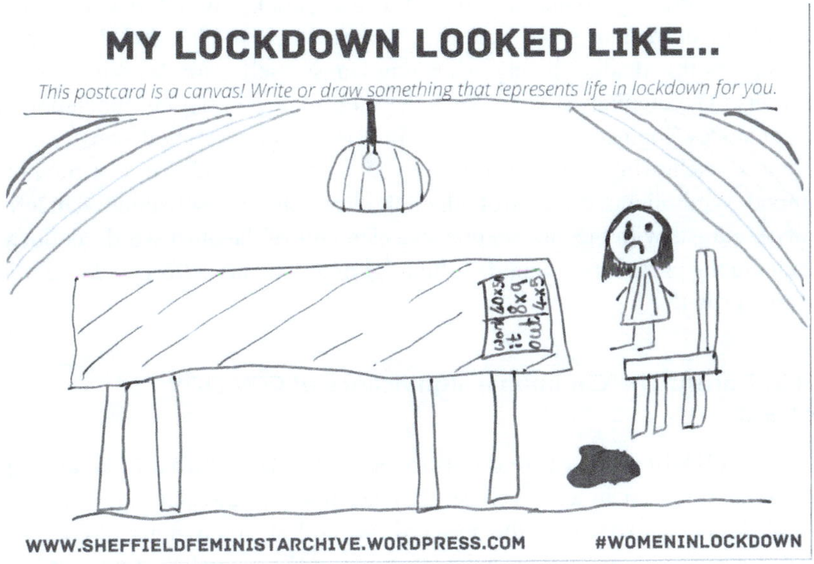

FIGURE 7.5 Anonymous. Postcard #7, Sheffield Feminist Archive, 2021–2022.

"carefully developed routines have been disrupted; support networks have disintegrated; and parents have been asked to do a job that trained teachers find challenging."[18] Christy Moran Craft and Jo Maseberg-Tomlinson define this added pressure as a "second shift,"[19] wherein childcare and housework function as a second, equally demanding job. The postcards, collectively, amplify this theme, curating a feminist narrative of struggle—what archival scholars describes as the collective articulation of multiple, overlapping individual experiences during the pandemic.[20] By curating and displaying such submissions, the archivists construct a feminist account of the pandemic—one that reveals how lockdowns exacerbated gendered inequalities in labor, making visible the impossible expectations placed on women as both workers and caregivers.

In contrast, other postcards express a tenuous contentment in life's small pleasures. In Postcard #9, the participant lists daily tasks as a means of grounding herself: "Studying for exams, Making use of the garden, Baking, Working out, Grateful to be with family (not living alone)."[21] Centered on the page, this organized list delineates both the structured routine and the monotony, each task an anchor against uncertainty. The final entry lands on a note of gratitude, a quiet assertion of resilience. As Sara Ahmed reminds us, crisis requires "a willingness to keep going despite or even because of what we come up against"—a feminist practice of perseverance.[22]

Archiving these postcards preserves women's pandemic experiences as historical artifacts, offering a window into the textures of daily lives during a crisis, from moments of despair to small victories. Postcard #22 in Carousel 2 (Figure 7.6) encapsulates this duality, listing "Cleaning House, Self Care, Working Freelance, Creativity, Developing Skills!, Writing + Journaling"[24] before concluding with "Personal Development."[23] The latter phrase is written in printed, square, geometric letters, eschewing rounded forms. Even the "o" is rendered as a rhombus or diamond, symbolizing the controlled, methodical nature of self-improvement. This choice contrasts with the more expressive elements of the other words, deliberately distancing the phrase from fluidity—highlighting structure, effort, and discipline in personal growth.

Still in Transit: The Communal Significance of COVID-19 Postcards

These COVID-19 postcards return us to Derrida's claim: "what I like about postcards is that even if in an envelope, they are made to circulate like an open but illegible letter" (12). He calls the postcard "so modest, anonymous, offered, stereotyped, 'retro'—and absolutely indecipherable" (47). COVID-19 postcards share this paradox. They are simple objects that resist final interpretation: "letters open, but like crypts" (53), exposing fragments that are both personal and encrypted. Like Derrida's illegible postcards, the Sheffield Feminist Archive COVID-19 postcards have no fixed meaning. Public and private, they attempt communication but

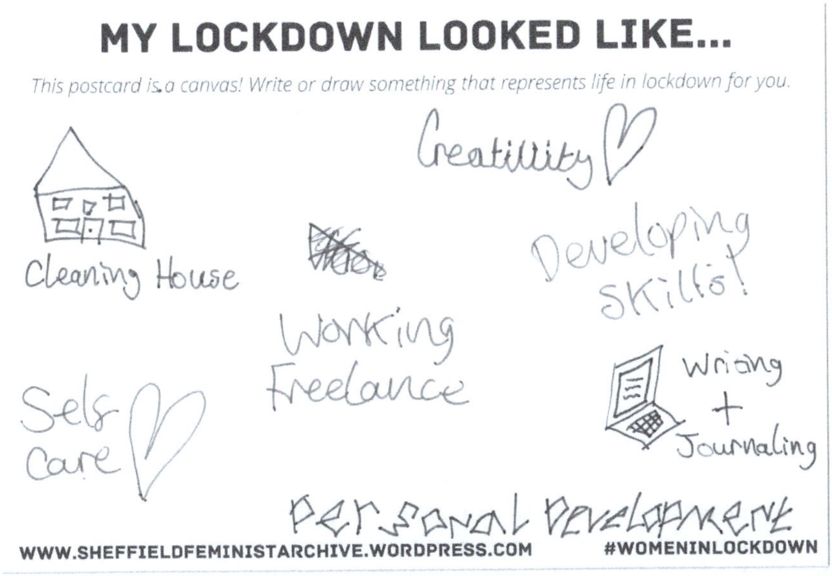

FIGURE 7.6 Anonymous. Postcard #22 in Carousel 2, Sheffield Feminist Archive, 2021–2022.

never fully arrive at a stable meaning. Their brevity heightens this instability: in capturing crisis, loss, or resilience in a few lines or images, they leave gaps—traces of an experience that resist articulation. As Derrida writes, they are "abandoned to an anonymous third-party, a neutral machinery that supposedly leads the message to its destination" (35).

Once submitted, these postcards enter an uncertain archival system, curated by archivists and interpreted by future readers. Like letters or diaries, they outlive their creators, detaching from original contexts. Meaning stays in flux, shaped by archival framing, reader assumptions, and changing historical understandings in which they are read. The postcards resist closure, embodying memory's instability. Yet, this instability is their value: as open-ended artifacts, they invite reinterpretation and keep the pandemic's lived experiences alive and shifting.

Where Derrida's postcards move through unknown postal hands, these COVID-19 postcards move through the hands of community archivists and researchers—each reshaping meaning in the act of reading. Derrida calls this process "terrifying": an attempt "to make [the message] indecipherable without compromising its making its way" (35). COVID-19 postcards travel through a similarly uncertain regime—linguistic, historical, emotional. They document by fragmentation, exposed to reinterpretation. Meaning is not merely deferred, but always unstable, questioning the notion of fixed documentation and exposing the unresolved nature of transmission itself.

The Sheffield archive's open-ended prompt—"What did my Lockdown look like . . ."—frames the project as both preservation and inquiry. The act of participating in the pandemic postcard project does, indeed, create a feminist community: the call explicitly solicits women's voices, and the project's mandate is grounded in feminist principles of care, inclusion, and everyday experience. That community is constituted not only by the archivists who solicit and curate the postcards but also by the women who write and submit them. Meanwhile, the postcard format is both liberating and limiting. It encourages concise, focused responses not always present in longer writing forms. Its brevity and open prompt invite diversity yet also steer contributors within certain expressive boundaries. Some may find the form unappealing—too restrictive, too plain, lacking in aesthetic richness. Still, these constraints prompted spontaneous and reflective insights that may risk oversimplifying but also distill emotion under pressure.

These postcard self-portraits offer catharsis for their creators—emotional release amid stress. They articulate which might remain unspoken in family and domestic contexts. The disclosures of increased alcohol or drug use, abuse, loneliness, depression, and loss, as depicted in these self-portraits, demonstrate how the postcards channeled the darker truths perhaps too difficult to express within the claustrophobic confines of domestic space. During the pandemic, many women struggled between caregiving demands and conflicted feelings about self-care, often seen as selfish. As cathartic self-portraits, these postcards are also ghostly, representing the ephemeral moments, even taboos, representations of women who may never have the chance to fully claim these experiences with their names attached. Yet through these postcards, their presence is still felt in the collective memory. Even post-COVID-19, these self-portrait "ghosts" persist through writing and drawing, existing between memory and history, haunting the archive, and quietly but powerfully contributing to the larger pandemic narrative.

In the Pandemic Postcards project, these artifacts are both personal and communal. Traditionally intimate, the postcard here becomes public intimacy, contributing to a shared record. The archive becomes a space where personal stories—of sacrifice, frustration, solidarity, adaptation—are woven into collective memory. Submitting these postcards is a feminist act, insisting that women's pandemic experiences are worth collecting, reading, and remembering.

By being preserved and actively integrated into the archive, these postcards transcend individual testimonies and contribute to a process of collaborative memory-building. The archive itself functions as a space where personal accounts resonate within the context of a larger collective experience. Even when postcards are not directly addressed to others, their inclusion in the archive transforms them into acts of community documentation, reflecting a shared social dialogue. This communal aspect of the archive extends beyond preserving personal experiences: it helps shape how these experiences are interpreted within the broader historical and social narrative of the pandemic. Through this process, the archive becomes more than a passive repository; it is a site of active community-building, where individual testimonies are solicited and interwoven into a collective historical record—one that reflects not only the diversity of experiences but also the common threads that bind them. It ultimately illuminates the feminist archive's active role in constructing a feminist history of the pandemic, while also legitimizing its own importance as an institution engaged in shaping the public memory of COVID-19.

Accompanying its deeply affective content as a catharsis for the creator, the materiality of the postcard self-portraits as surviving archival objects plays a crucial role in preserving pandemic experiences. For those visiting the archive, these postcards preserve what archival theorist Marika Cifor calls "liveliness"—material traces of lived reality that can still be felt years and decades later. She writes, "Through the lens of liveliness, the relations of archival records, the space of the archives, and the other actors (human and non-human) involved can be understood as moving, changeable, and interrelated constructions."[24] This perspective is particularly relevant to COVID-19 testimonials, where personal artifacts—postcards, handwritten notes, or visual sketches—preserve affective and bodily traces that remain active in the archive.

Themes of loneliness and isolation appear frequently in the Sheffield archives, as well as narratives of anger and abuse. In postcard #11 (see Figure 7.3), a woman surrounded by family still expresses a deep sense of solitude. Postcard #65 similarly depicts a woman tucked in bed with the handwritten caption "rotting in bed," surrounded by headphones, an open book, and an uneaten piece of toast.[25] These visual and textual self-narratives highlight the pandemic's emotional tool, particularly on women, who make up about 70% of the global health workforce and often faced extreme pressures with little institutional support.[26] While the Pandemic Postcard collection includes self-representations that acknowledge both resilience and exhaustion, images of quasi-heroism are largely absent in the Sheffield project.

Thus, we must return to earlier distinction embedded in the creation of pandemic postcards. During World War I, soldiers wrote postcards and personal diaries and created trench art, much of which remained in private family collections and was only later incorporated into institutional archives. In other words, these objects were made in the moment but were only recognized as public archival material later. In contrast, the women's pandemic postcards in Sheffield were directly solicited, making their archival preservation almost certain upon submission. As forms of life writing, these postcards document personal pandemic experiences, memories, and stories. In this sense, self-writing and self-drawing—particularly when explicitly invited—take on an even more cathartic role for the creator.

Ultimately, women's pandemic postcards, like many documents and records, serve a dual function: they document lived experiences while also enabling the processing of trauma.[27] Here, the archival act of soliciting self-portraits during COVID-19 creates a space for both catharsis and the creation of testimonial artifacts. The community-based nature of the project deepens this process, transforming it into an act of collective remembrance—one that not only preserves history but also reshapes personal and communal narratives in its wake.

Notes

1 Postcard #47, 2021–2022, Pandemic Postcards, Sheffield Feminist Archive, https://sheffieldfeministarchive.wordpress.com/women-in-lockdown/pandemic-postcards/#jp-carousel-2696.
2 Postcard #45, 2021–2022, Pandemic Postcards, Sheffield Feminist Archive, https://sheffieldfeministarchive.wordpress.com/women-in-lockdown/pandemic-postcards/#jp-carousel-2695.
3 Sheffield Feminist Archives, Community Archive and Heritage Group, accessed February 21, 2025, https://www.communityarchives.org.uk/content/organisation/sheffield-feminist-archive.
4 For a timeline of the pandemic, see J. Michael Ryan, "Timeline of the COVID-19 Pandemic," in *COVID-19: Individual Rights and Community Responsibilities* (Routledge, 2023), xvii–xxxviii.
5 Lucy Brownson et al., "Autonomous Archives: Reframing Feminist Heritage in the Context of COVID-19," in *Routledge International Handbook of Heritage and Gender*, ed. Jenna C. Ashton (Routledge, 2025), 398–413.
6 We are also reminded that postcards were traditionally linked to the upheaval of wars, given that soldiers during World War I, for example, were encouraged to write to families before major battles. This meant that a soldier sending a postcard as a sign of life to their loved ones might, in fact, be wounded or dead by the time of its arrival.
7 Postcard #14, 2021–2022, Pandemic Postcards, Sheffield Feminist Archive, https://sheffieldfeministarchive.wordpress.com/women-in-lockdown/pandemic-postcards/#jp-carousel-4042.
8 Sidonie Smith and Julia Watson, *Reading Autobiography Now: An Updated Guide for Interpreting Life Narratives*, 3rd ed. (Minneapolis, MN: University of Minnesota Press, 2024), 104.
9 William Whyte, "*Seven Lives from Mass Observation: Britain in the Late Twentieth Century* by James Hinton, Book Review," *Modern British History* 28, no. 3 (September 2017): 480–88, https://doi.org/10.1093/tcbh/hwx001.
10 Erving Goffman, "On Face-Work: An Analysis of Ritual Elements in Social Interaction," *Psychiatry* 18, no. 3 (August 1955): 213–31, www.tandfonline.com/doi/abs/10.1080/00332747.1955.11023008, https://doi.org/10.1080/00332747.1955.11023008.
11 Michael Humphrey and Elias Gbadamosi, "The 'Imagined Author': Contingent Selves in an Anonymous Life Writing Subreddit," *Journal of Comparative Literature & Aesthetics* 44, no. 4 (2022): 164.
12 Yasmin B. Kafai et al., "Your Second Selves: Avatar Designs and Identity Play," *Games and Culture* 1, no. 5 (2010): 26.
13 Postcard #11, 2021–2022, Pandemic Postcards, Sheffield Feminist Archive, https://sheffieldfeministarchive.wordpress.com/women-in-lockdown/pandemic-postcards/#jp-carousel-4040.
14 Breanne Fahs, "'He's Thinking About Sex, I'm Thinking About Survival': Women's Sexual, Domestic, and Emotional Labor During the COVID-19 Pandemic," in *Creative Resilience and COVID-19*, ed. Irene Gammel and Jason Wang (Routledge, 2022), 70–81.
15 Hillary L. Chute, *Graphic Women: Life Narrative and Contemporary Comics* (Columbia University Press, 2010).
16 Postcard #26, 2021–2022, Pandemic Postcards, Sheffield Feminist Archive, https://sheffieldfeministarchive.wordpress.com/women-in-lockdown/pandemic-postcards/#jp-carousel-4077.
17 Postcard #7, 2021–2022, Pandemic Postcards, Sheffield Feminist Archive, https://sheffieldfeministarchive.wordpress.com/women-in-lockdown/pandemic-postcards/#jp-carousel-4031.

18 Kathryn Asbury et al., "How Is COVID-19 Affecting the Mental Health of Children with Special Educational Needs and Disabilities and Their Families?" *Journal of Autism and Developmental Disorder* 51 (2021): 1772–80, https://doi.org/10.1007/s10803-020-04577-2.

19 Christy Moran Craft and Jo Maseberg-Tomlinson quoted in Dorothea Bowyer et al., "Academic Mothers, Professional Identity and COVID-19: Feminist Reflections on Career Cycles, Progression and Practice," *Gender, Work & Organization* 29, no. 1 (2022): 311.

20 Marika Cifor and Stacy Wood, "Critical Feminism in the Archives," *Journal of Critical Library and Information Studies* 1, no. 2 (2017): 10.

21 Postcard #9, 2021–2022, Pandemic Postcards, Sheffield Feminist Archive, https://sheffieldfeministarchive.wordpress.com/women-in-lockdown/pandemic-postcards/#jp-carousel-4038.

22 Sara Ahmed, "Introduction: Bringing Feminist Theory Home," in *Living a Feminist Life* (Duke University Press, 2017), 1–18.

23 Postcard #22 in Carousel 2, 2021–2022, Pandemic Postcards, Sheffield Feminist Archive, https://sheffieldfeministarchive.wordpress.com/women-in-lockdown/pandemic-postcards/#jp-carousel-2677.

24 Marika Cifor, "Stains and Remains: Liveliness, Materiality, and the Archival Lives of Queer Bodies," in *Archives and New Modes of Feminist Research*, ed. Maryanne Dever (Routledge, 2020), 6.

25 Postcard #65, 2021–2022, Pandemic Postcards, Sheffield Feminist Archive, https://sheffieldfeministarchive.wordpress.com/women-in-lockdown/pandemic-postcards/#jp-carousel-4121.

26 Remya Lathabhavan and Prabir Chandra Padhy, *Community Mental Health and Well-Being in the New Normal* (IGI Global, 2023).

27 Diana Taylor, "Trauma in the Archive," in *Feeling Photography*, ed. Elspeth H. Brown and Thy Phu (Duke University Press, 2014), 239–51.

Bibliography

Ahmed, Sara. "Introduction: Bringing Feminist Theory Home." In *Living a Feminist Life*, 1–18. Duke University Press, 2016. https://doi.org/10.2307/j.ctv11g9836.4.

Asbury, Kathryn, Laura Fox, Emre Deniz, Aimee Code, and Umar Toseeb. "How Is COVID-19 Affecting the Mental Health of Children with Special Educational Needs and Disabilities and Their Families?" *Journal of Autism and Developmental Disorders* 51, no. 5 (2021): 1772–80. https://doi.org/10.1007/s10803-020-04577-2.

Bowyer, Dorothea, Milissa Deitz, Anne Jamison, Chloe E. Taylor, Erika Gyengesi, Jaime Ross, Hollie Hammond, Anita Eseosa Ogbeide, and Tinashe Dune. "Academic Mothers, Professional Identity and COVID-19: Feminist Reflections on Career Cycles, Progression and Practice." *Gender, Work & Organization* 29, no. 1 (2022): 309–41. https://doi.org/10.1111/gwao.12750.

Chute, Hillary L. *Graphic Women: Life Narrative and Contemporary Comics*. New York: Columbia University Press, 2010.

Cifor, Marika. "Stains and Remains: Liveliness, Materiality, and the Archival Lives of Queer Bodies." *Australian Feminist Studies* 32, no. 91–92 (2017): 5–21. https://doi.org/10.1080/08164649.2017.1357014.

Cifor, Marika, and Stacy Wood. "Critical Feminism in the Archives." *Journal of Critical Library and Information Studies* 1, no. 2 (2017): 1–27. https://doi.org/10.24242/jclis.v1i2.27.

Fahs, Breanne. "'He's Thinking About Sex, I'm Thinking About Survival' Women's Sexual, Domestic, and Emotional Labor During the COVID-19 Pandemic." In *Creative*

Resilience and COVID-19, edited by Jason Wang and Irene Gammel, 1st ed., 70–81. Routledge, 2022. https://doi.org/10.4324/9781003213536-9.

Humphrey, Michael, and Elias Gbadamosi. "The 'Imagined Author': Contingent Selves in an Anonymous Life Writing Subreddit." *Journal of Comparative Literature & Aesthetics* 44, no. 4 (2022): 164–74.

Kafai, Yasmin B., Deborah A. Fields, and Melissa S. Cook. "Your Second Selves: Player-Designed Avatars." *Games and Culture* 5, no. 1 (2010): 23–42. https://doi.org/10.1177/1555412009351260.

Lathabhavan, Remya, and Prabir Chandra Padhy. *Community Mental Health and Well-Being in the New Normal*, 1st ed. Hershey, PA: IGI Global, 2023. https://doi.org/10.4018/978-1-6684-7221-7.

Ryan, J. Michael. *COVID-19: Individual Rights and Community Responsibilities*. Edited by J. Michael Ryan, 1st ed. New York: Routledge, 2023. https://doi.org/10.4324/9781003302643.

Sheffield Feminist Archive. "Pandemic Postcards." Sheffield Feminist Archive, March 20, 2025.

Sheffield Feminist Archive. "Sheffield Feminist Archive." Community Archives and Heritage Group, March 16, 2021. https://www.communityarchives.org.uk/content/organisation/sheffield-feminist-archive.

Smith, Sidonie, and Julia Watson. *Reading Autobiography Now: An Updated Guide for Interpreting Life Narratives*, 3rd ed. Minneapolis: University of Minnesota Press, 2024.

Taylor, Diana. "Trauma in the Archive." In *Feeling Photography*, edited by Elspeth H. Brown and Thy Phu, 239–51. Duke University Press, 2014. https://doi.org/10.2307/j.ctv11319fq.15.

Whyte, William. "Review of Seven Lives from Mass Observation: Britain in the Late Twentieth Century, by James Hinton." *20th Century British History* 28, no. 3 (2017): 480–81. https://doi.org/10.1093/tcbh/hwx001.

PART III

Life Writing Through Media Ecologies

8

FRAGMENTS OF CARE

Hassan Akkad's Refugee Testimony in a Time of Crisis

Ana Belén Martínez García

I have long been drawn to questions of identity—how it is shaped, performed, and often contested—particularly through the lenses of socio-cultural, gender, and performativity studies. My work has led me to explore life narratives that bear witness to human rights struggles, especially those that foreground empathy as a political and ethical force, both online and offline. Much of this work focuses on life writing as a tool of testimony: a way for vulnerable youth and women to resist the reductive labels that so often define them. By writing about refugee activists and how emotions regarding their plight surface in public discourse, it becomes clear how vulnerability—especially in contexts of forced displacement—can be reimagined as a source of strength. These questions came into sharp focus for me during the pandemic, when I was deeply moved by the story of filmmaker and activist Hassan Akkad, a young Syrian refugee whose experience unsettled many of the categories I thought I understood.

When the COVID-19 pandemic struck the United Kingdom in March 2020, Hassan Akkad found himself in a state of precarious limbo. As a refugee awaiting a decision on his asylum claim, he was already grappling with the uncertainties and hostilities of displacement. The pandemic's lockdowns deepened this isolation, amplifying the struggles of being an unwanted, unacknowledged individual. In the midst of this intensified vulnerability, Akkad published *Hope Not Fear* (2021), a memoir that brought the conditions of marginalization into sudden public view.[1] His voice and the voices of others pushed to society's edges reached audiences through viral circulation on social media. What struck me was how his writing held together multiple forms of precariousness—refugee status, systemic neglect, and the exhaustion of frontline work—without collapsing into each other. *Hope Not Fear* can be read as a testimonial text, a form of life writing that bears witness to upheaval, injustice, and hope.[2] Testimonial narratives—memoirs, oral histories,

DOI: 10.4324/9781003735595-12

public statements—offer firsthand insights into lived crises and function as acts of advocacy, fostering empathy and demanding accountability. Akkad's first-person account, the "I," that speaks to the reader is not only personal but also politically situated—a witness to systemic violence: the Syrian revolution, wrongful detention, torture, forced migration, racism, and a global pandemic. His story opens a space for relational ethics and shared vulnerability.

What is especially striking is how the narrative invites connection. Inspired by ideas about relationality and care, we can see how Akkad's voice gains strength through various encounters—with readers, users, audiences, and co-sufferers. His memoir assembles what might be called an interhuman network of care—where the entanglements of personal and collective struggle produce new, sometimes fragile, solidarities. This is not a story shaped by timidity or defeat. It is a record of people reaching toward one another under pressure and of hope as a deliberate orientation.

While some studies have explored the impact of prolonged uncertainty and immobility on asylum seekers' mental health,[3] the lived experience of this trauma—layered atop previous displacements—remains undertheorized.[4] *Hope Not Fear* might at first seem to belong to the wave of COVID-19 "diaries" that proliferated during lockdown as discussed in this volume (see Chapters 2 and 6). But its scope is different. Akkad's memoir does not isolate the pandemic as a singular crisis; it threads it into a longer arc of political violence and resistance.

These strands resist separation. Together they construct the identity of the narrator-activist, whose testimony transforms personal survival into a call for collective resistance.

Testimony and Assemblage Theory

Akkad's layered, relational form of self-narration echoes the workings of what Sidonie Smith and Julia Watson describe as the testimonial "I" in *Reading Autobiography Now* (2024). For them, the "I" is never fixed or autonomous; it is shaped through context, through contact with others, through the pressures and urgencies of its time, emphasizing its construction through social forces.[5] In testimonial writing, the self is constantly negotiated—through memory, through the demands of political life, and through the need to speak not only for oneself but also sometimes on behalf of a community. The "I" here becomes porous, unstable, and responsive—qualities that feel especially familiar in the wake of a pandemic that upended certainties and exposed long-standing inequalities.

Philosopher Jane Bennett offers a different but complementary lens. In *Vibrant Matter: A Political Ecology of Things* (2010), she argues for an extended sense of agency—one that includes not only humans but also nonhuman entities—objects, infrastructures, and systems.[6] For Bennett, power is created through assemblages: webs of human and nonhuman elements that act together. These assemblages resist the idea of isolated action; they show how influence and change are distributed across bodies, spaces, and materials. Much like the testimonial "I," the assemblage does not concentrate power in one place. Instead, it maps how relations themselves do the work—how the world is shaped by encounters between people, viruses, machines, and stories.

This framework helps clarify the stakes of writing through the pandemic. As J. Michael Ryan and Serena Nanda argue in *COVID-19: Social Inequalities and Human Possibilities*, the virus doesn't operate outside of society—it is embedded in it.[7] It interacts with policies, access to care, economic systems, and histories of oppression. Like Bennett's assemblage, the pandemic exposes how deeply entangled we are with forces beyond our control. And like the testimonial "I," it demands that we stay attuned to how personal experience is always threaded through larger structures.

Akkad's memoir displays this entanglement. His narrative refuses easy separations between the personal and the political, between grief and resistance, between the body and the system. What emerges is not a story of isolated crisis, but of ongoing struggle, shaped by forces that cannot be contained by one individual. And perhaps this is what makes testimony important now: not only its capacity to document but also its insistence that we are connected—to others, to history, and to the world we continue to shape together.

Testimony and Activism: Hassan Akkad's Journey

Akkad's memoir opens with childhood memories, not out of nostalgia, but to expose the harsh realities of growing up in Syria under Bashar al-Assad's regime, where "human rights" were nonexistent.[8] From early indoctrination at school[9] to military training at age 12,[10] he recalls a "system of lies and intimidation" designed to instill fear and obedience.[11] Unflinchingly self-aware, Akkad admits he and his friends were "sexist" and "xenophobic,"[12] and "often homophobic, too."[13] These confessions frame the activist he becomes, driven by a belief that access to information can dismantle prejudice: "People are afraid of what they don't understand."[14] This realization leads him to teaching and later to documenting injustice as a filmmaker.

Akkad's activism and filmmaking mirror the rapid escalation of the Arab Spring in Syria beginning in 2011.[15] Participating in demonstrations and recording atrocities, he vindicates the importance of citizen journalism,[16] emphasizing the necessity of first-person accounts in exposing authoritarian violence. However, his work leads to multiple escapes before he is eventually detained and tortured:

> The secret police . . . were trained to kill,. . . surefooted and lethal,. . . beating us, going for our faces and chests . . . the blows rained down. I immediately felt I was being hurt, . . . bones . . . breaking . . . I could no longer protect my face. "You want freedom," they shouted. "Here's your freedom."[17]

This brutal scene underscores how state violence during the Arab Spring was not just repressive but calculated—a strategy aimed at erasing identity and extinguishing collective will.

Akkad's subsequent imprisonment, marked by extreme abuse, only deepens the trauma:

> We were stacked up on top of each other, like sardines in a tin. . . . [The guard] jumped on my chest, over and over again with his thick-soled military shoes. The full force of his body . . . cracked several of my ribs . . . I felt a searing pain, like nothing I had felt before.[18]

Stripped, humiliated, and beaten, Akkad reflects: "I still live with the legacy of the physical injuries—but my mind was also never the same. The young man I had been was gone forever."[19] This kind of psychic disintegration recalls the disorientation of the COVID-19 pandemic, where selfhood was similarly fractured by institutional neglect, overcrowded hospitals, and the sheer vulnerability of the body. In both cases, care and control became entangled, and resistance seemed nearly impossible.

After surviving and nearly losing his leg to infection, Akkad attempts to return to teaching but remains under constant surveillance and is eventually detained again. This time, the violence he endures is even more destructive: "the abuse completely shattered the self-image I'd developed, as an Arab man, forever."[20] Akkad later learns that sexual abuse is part of a deliberate strategy used by the regime to break its opposition: "What seemed random was most likely anything but. The regime didn't like members of the opposition who were like me. Young, bright, dynamic, professionally successful. They set about systematically breaking us."[21] His decision to flee to Europe is not rushed but born from a life in limbo, denied basic rights in neighboring countries. In an intimate tone, Akkad reveals his ultimate motivation: "security isn't just about being safe from imminent death. It's also about having a future, options, the autonomy to build a life of your choosing."[22] Here, Akkad redefines security not as mere survival but as the ability to shape one's own future with autonomy and choice. His reflection challenges the idea that safety is simply the absence of danger, arguing instead that true security comes from having the freedom to build a meaningful life.

The journey across the Mediterranean in a dinghy changes Akkad's perspective. He realizes his previous criticisms of displaced people were misguided. This led him to document the abuses he saw for what would become *Exodus: Our Journey to Europe*,[23] a BAFTA-awarded documentary aired on BBC2. Akkad's memoir challenges the media's often politicized and biased portrayal of asylum seekers. He seeks to dismantle misconceptions:

> There is rhetoric that refugees come to drain benefits . . . bankrupting Britain. They really aren't. All sorts of things might be bringing this country to

> economic ruin, but it definitely isn't the fault of the most vulnerable . . . . And all I have ever wanted to do is to make a contribution and to work.[24]

While awaiting resolution of his asylum claim, Akkad becomes more open about his past, reconstructing his traumatic experience not only for his own healing but to help others:

> We shape our societies through the stories we tell about ourselves. . . . Not being able to speak your truth . . . is nothing short of dehumanizing. . . . by articulating what had happened to me, offering up my version of events, I was shaping my own, often brutal and apparently arbitrary, experiences into something cohesive and meaningful.[25]

His words stand for those of the silenced who cannot tell their story. At the same time, Akkad harnesses empathy to illustrate the transformative power of testimony.[26] He rejects the notion that refugees and migrants seek mere compassion: "People don't want sympathy, they want opportunity. Refugees don't want people to pity them. They want internships, job opportunities, concrete offers."[27] This reflects a broader need shared by vulnerable people who seek attention and recognition instead of pity[28] and applies to Akkad's COVID-19 experience as a refugee in London.

Vulnerable Volunteering: COVID-19, Life Writing, and Testimony

As Hassan Akkad's memoir offers a personal testimony of his experience volunteering in a COVID-19 ward, his narrative provides ample scope for reflection on the ethical obligations inherent in life writing during the pandemic. In what he describes as "The Red Zone"[29] of Whipps Cross Hospital,[30] Akkad encounters the convergence of paralyzing fear, a dearth of information, and the quiet heroism of people working without adequate resources. His testimony extends beyond his own experience; it gives voice to those who cannot speak for themselves—the patients and colleagues who died unseen and unheard, and to those whose exhaustion and grief never made headlines.

Akkad's memories carry both the disorientation of a volunteer thrown into chaos and the determination to make that experience meaningful. The "flimsy kit" used by medical workers—at once "precious" and alarmingly "scarce"—emerges as a symbol of the larger instability he faces.[31] Confusing, frequently shifting protocols only deepen that uncertainty. These moments are not unique to him but part of a broader, shared vulnerability that COVID-19 life writing attempts to express: not just personal toll, but the systemic failures that shaped it.

His narrative gains force from its focus on others. When he recounts a man begging to see his dying mother—refused by a nurse for safety reasons[32]—Akkad's empathy becomes a point of connection, not just with the man, but with readers too. He doesn't offer easy answers or heroic gestures, only the quiet truth of being unable to help, of wanting to do more. It's in that moment that care takes on a deeper meaning. Rather than physical intervention, care becomes, as María Puig de la Bellacasa suggests, a political and ethical orientation—a commitment to staying attuned to others, even in powerlessness.[33]

Akkad's writing takes up this form of care as a relational and vulnerable stance. His memoir asks readers to be affected—to feel what it meant to live, work, and fear in the COVID ward—and to question how such suffering was handled by the institutions meant to protect us. Testimony here becomes a form of collective reckoning. In continuing the work he began as a citizen journalist in Syria, Akkad shifts his lens from exposing authoritarian brutality to confronting quieter but no less destructive forms of systemic neglect. His voice joins the long tradition of testimonial writing, where first-person narratives speak for those silenced and call others to listen with care and responsibility.

Reclaiming the Right to Be Seen and Heard: Collective Testimony in Akkad's Memoir

It is not enough to simply testify to the injustices of the healthcare system and the unmet needs of the ill and their families. Akkad does not isolate his own story; he places it among others, highlighting the collective efforts of those deemed powerless, yet crucial to the country's survival during a time of crisis. Akkad's viral tweets—first a photograph, then a video—urged the government to support those working in the National Health Service (NHS). As his visibility increased, Akkad began to speak not only for himself but also for his colleagues and friends, many of whom could not speak English. In doing so, he brought together the experiences of silenced frontline workers, whose dedication has been consistently overlooked, much like their social and documentation statuses.

Importantly, Akkad advocates for the dignity of care workers who are typically unrecognized—those whose labor is vital yet overshadowed by the more celebrated roles of doctors and nurses. In a humorous yet profoundly ethical statement, Akkad reflects on the class divisions within the hospital, writing:

> Whipps Cross started to remind me of the Titanic. A vast ship, with the upper classes—the doctors and nurses—on the top floors and the lower classes—cleaners like me, porters, ward hosts, the Serco staff—on the ground floor. The class divisions were clear and yet it was swiftly obvious how deeply reliant everyone in the building was on those who worked on the lower deck.[34]

Akkad's metaphor of the Titanic brings home how stark those divides felt on the ground, even as everyone relied on one another to survive. These workers, many of whom were invisible before the pandemic, were also hidden during the very moment they risked their lives for those who disregarded them. Class and race intertwine in Akkad's testimony, drawing attention to the ways these workers' humanity is denied by systemic neglect, echoing historical injustices like apartheid or Jim Crow laws:

> Such an obvious separation wasn't what I anticipated . . . Or that a disproportionate number of ethnic minority workers would die of coronavirus. It was striking how the doctors and management team at the hospital were predominantly white, while my new colleagues weren't.[35]

He shows how this separation and neglect echo the systemic racism and segregation of the past, not only persisting during the pandemic but also intensifying.

In this sense, Akkad not only shares his own experience but also becomes an advocate for the unseen—those workers whose stories rarely surface. His posts on Twitter and Instagram, shared in the hope of raising awareness, create space for readers to become witnesses and assemble these fragmented stories. As Smith and Watson suggest, this mobilization of identity—where individual voices become platforms for political claims—is common to testimonial narratives,[36] which here underscores Akkad's broader effort to push for recognition and rights for the workers whose labor is so often overlooked.

Rather than simply recounting what happened, Akkad's narrative urges readers to see differently. His storytelling weaves together individual "I"s into a larger narrative, creating what Smith and Watson describe as "fluid assemblages."[37] It is the shared agency of this assemblage—where human actors, materials, and systems intersect—that encourages readers to see beyond the isolated experience and recognize the full range of contributions from all of the involved factors. As this collective testimony unfolds, the voices join together to reconstruct the larger experience of pandemic and post-pandemic society.

Sociologist Sean Creaven explores how British exceptionalism and neoliberalism compounded the crisis, especially for those working in social care.[38] He notes that post-Brexit immigration policies threaten the status of these essential workers, many of whom come from non-white ethnic minority communities. Despite this, migrant workers—often underpaid and overburdened—continue to support a system that neglects them. Akkad reflects on the vital role played by immigrants in the NHS: "it was quickly clear to me how much the ward was held up by immigrants. Most of the porters, cleaners, healthcare assistants had come from other countries."[39] Akkad's memoir cuts through the abstractions of the faceless "hero,"[40] offering instead a more grounded recognition of every worker—regardless of their background or status—as someone who deserves to be seen and heard. By collecting the stories of those around him, he validates their human rights, recognizing their intrinsic worth and dismantling the erasure imposed by a system that fails to acknowledge their humanity. Through this act of collective storytelling, Akkad lays bare how essential these workers are to any functioning idea of care, creating an assemblage that reflects the diverse, interconnected fabric of post-pandemic Britain.

Looking Ahead: Hope for the Future?

The COVID-19 pandemic laid bare deep societal inequalities, revealing how structural divisions in race, class, gender, and sexuality remain entrenched, despite the virus's indiscriminate nature. As Ryan and Nanda point out, pandemics expose these fractures more starkly than most crises.[41] While the virus did not discriminate, it emphasized just how much society does. In this context, Hassan Akkad directly challenged any comforting notion of the pandemic as "the greatest equalizer." Instead, he asserts that the crisis "exposed the inequalities that exist in our society. Covid will go, but these injustices won't."[42] For these injustices to be addressed, Akkad insists, we must act. Just as his work as a citizen journalist in Syria exposed authoritarian violence, his role as a healthcare worker in London compelled him to speak out against systemic prejudice in the British healthcare system. His message is direct and personal: awareness must lead to responsibility. This simple yet forceful claim is echoed by a broader theme of the pandemic—its dual capacity to reveal both suffering and possibility. While the crisis exposed deep vulnerabilities, it also opened space for transformation, both personal and collective.

Akkad's story does not unfold neatly, and neither does trauma or upheaval. With its non-linear structure, his narrative shows how pain resists coherence while also demonstrating the power of collective action. His testimony invites us to reconnect with the raw emotions of this time, making us active participants in the emotional journey shared by healthcare workers and others on the frontlines. Their courage, despite immense personal risks, forces us to reconsider what we mean by human strength and endurance. As healthcare workers persevered through physical and psychological hardships, they exemplified the strength needed to endure the most difficult circumstances.

Akkad's account as a migrant healthcare worker also directly confronts the stereotypes that often reduce or erase such lives. His witnessing—both online and offline—helps dismantle these damaging portrayals at a time when such voices are crucial. His call to action is not abstract: it's in invitation to participate. "We're all interconnected. Our humanity unites us,"[43] he writes, underscoring the interdependence that holds the promise of a more just future. In the face of the pandemic's harsh realities, Akkad's activism shows readers that hope is not just an abstract ideal but a call to action. By fostering empathy and unity, we can shape a more equitable world, where the fragility of human existence is met with solidarity rather than division. This vision of connection—both pressing and deeply personal—offers a foundation for a hopeful future, one where readers, as empathic witnesses, help drive the change Akkad calls for.

Acknowledgments: This work is part of Grant PID2022–137881NB-I00, "Re-orienting Assemblage Theory in Anglophone Literature and Culture" (RELY), led by Prof. Rosario Arias, funded by the Spanish Ministry of Science, Innovation and Universities MCIN/AEI/10.13039/501100011033 and co-funded by the European Regional Development Fund "A way of making Europe."

Notes

1 Hassan Akkad, *Hope Not Fear: Finding My Way from Refugee to Filmmaker, to NHS Hospital Cleaner and Activist* (London: Bluebird, 2021).
2 The edition used in this chapter is the paperback, which has a slightly different title: Hassan Akkad, *Hope Not Fear: Finding My Way from Refugee to Filmmaker and Activist* (London: Bluebird, 2023). All citations will thus refer to the 2023 edition.
3 Mattias De Backer et al., "'Their Lives Are Even More on Hold Now': Migrants' Experiences of Waiting and Immobility During the COVID-19 Pandemic," *Social & Cultural Geography* 24, no. 10 (2023): 1846–62; Noel B. Salazar, "Immobility: The Relational and Experiential Qualities of an Ambiguous Concept," *Transfers* 11, no. 3 (2021): 3–21.
4 Ana Belén Martínez García, "Memories of War and the COVID-19 Crisis in Spain," *Human Arenas* 4 (2021): 366–78.
5 Sidonie Smith and Julia Watson, *Reading Autobiography Now: An Updated Guide for Interpreting Life Narratives*, 3rd ed. (Minneapolis: University of Minnesota Press, 2024), 228.
6 Jane Bennett, *Vibrant Matter: A Political Ecology of Things* (Durham: Duke University Press, 2010).
7 J. Michael Ryan and Serena Nanda, *COVID-19: Social Inequalities and Human Possibilities* (Abingdon: Routledge, 2022).
8 Akkad, *Hope Not Fear*, 10.
9 Akkad, *Hope Not Fear*, 10.
10 Akkad, *Hope Not Fear*, 11.
11 Akkad, *Hope Not Fear*, 12.
12 Akkad, *Hope Not Fear*, 13.
13 Akkad, *Hope Not Fear*, 14.
14 Akkad, *Hope Not Fear*, 14.
15 The Arab Spring began in Tunisia on December 17, 2010, when Mohamed Bouazizi set himself on fire to protest police abuse and poverty. His act ignited uprisings across the Middle East and North Africa against authoritarian rule, corruption, and economic hardship, toppling leaders in Tunisia, Egypt, Libya, and Yemen. While some countries saw reforms, others, like Syria, descended into conflict and chaos, leaving a legacy of both hope and instability.
16 Akkad, *Hope Not Fear*, 44.
17 Akkad, *Hope Not Fear*, 47.
18 Akkad, *Hope Not Fear*, 49–50.
19 Akkad, *Hope Not Fear*, 51.
20 Akkad, *Hope Not Fear*, 97.
21 Akkad, *Hope Not Fear*, 103.
22 Akkad, *Hope Not Fear*, 116.
23 James Bluemel, dir., *Exodus: Our Journey to Europe* (Keo Films, 2016).
24 Akkad, *Hope Not Fear*, 193.
25 Akkad, *Hope Not Fear*, 195.
26 Suzanne Keen, "Strategic Empathizing: Techniques of Bounded, Ambassadorial, and Broadcast Narrative Empathy," *Deutsche Vierteljahrsschrift für Literaturwissenschaft und Geistesgeschichte* 82, no. 3 (2008): 477–93. Keen's article explores three types of narrative empathy: bounded empathy, which is confined to specific characters or events; ambassadorial empathy, which advocates for understanding others or social causes; and broadcast empathy, which aims to engage a broad audience for emotional or political impact. These forms are strategically used by authors to influence the reader's ethical engagement with the narrative and its broader social implications.
27 Akkad, *Hope Not Fear*, 201.

28 Rosalía Baena, "No Pity: Disability Memoirs and Narrative Empathy in Robert Murphy's *The Body Silent* and Reynolds Price's *A Whole New Life*," *Concentric: Literary and Cultural Studies* 42, no. 2 (2016): 65–83.
29 Akkad, *Hope Not Fear*, 4.
30 Founded as a military hospital during World War I, Whipps Cross Hospital is a large hospital in London, England. It is part of the Barts Health National Health Service (NHS) Trust.
31 Akkad, *Hope Not Fear*, 5.
32 Akkad, *Hope Not Fear*, 7.
33 Maria Puig de la Bellacasa, "Matters of Care in Technoscience: Assembling Neglected Things," *Social Studies of Science* 41, no. 1 (2011): 90. See also Maria Puig de la Bellacasa, *Matters of Care: Speculative Ethics in More than Human Worlds* (Minneapolis: University of Minnesota Press, 2017).
34 Akkad, *Hope Not Fear*, 245.
35 Akkad, *Hope Not Fear*, 245.
36 Smith and Watson, *Reading Autobiography Now*, 71.
37 Smith and Watson, *Reading Autobiography Now*, 100.
38 Sean Creaven, *The Pandemic in Britain: COVID-19, British Exceptionalism and Neoliberalism* (Abingdon: Routledge, 2023).
39 Akkad, *Hope Not Fear*, 7.
40 Sophie Hennekam, Jamie Ladge, and Yuliya Shymko, "From Zero to Hero: An Exploratory Study Examining Sudden Hero Status Among Nonphysician Health Care Workers During the COVID-19 Pandemic," *Journal of Applied Psychology* 105, no. 10 (2020): 1088–100.
41 J. Michael Ryan and Serena Nanda, *COVID-19: Social Inequalities and Human Possibilities* (Abingdon: Routledge, 2022).
42 Akkad, *Hope Not Fear*, 226.
43 Akkad, *Hope Not Fear*, 288.

Bibliography

Akkad, Hassan. *Hope Not Fear: Finding My Way from Refugee to Filmmaker and Activist*. London: Bluebird, 2023.

Akkad, Hassan. *Hope Not Fear: Finding My Way from Refugee to Filmmaker, to NHS Hospital Cleaner and Activist*. London: Bluebird, 2021.

Baena, Rosalía. "No Pity: Disability Memoirs and Narrative Empathy in Robert Murphy's *The Body Silent* and Reynolds Price's *A Whole New Life*." *Concentric: Literary and Cultural Studies* 42, no. 2 (2016): 65–83. https://doi.org/10.6240/concentric.lit.2016.42.2.05.

Bennett, Jane. *Vibrant Matter: A Political Ecology of Things*. Durham: Duke University Press, 2010.

Bluemel, James, dir. *Exodus: Our Journey to Europe*. Keo Films, 2016.

Creaven, Sean. *The Pandemic in Britain: COVID-19, British Exceptionalism and Neoliberalism*. Abingdon: Routledge, 2023.

De Backer, Mattias, Pascale Felten, Elisabeth Kirndörfer, Mieke Kox, and Robin Finlay. " 'Their Lives Are Even More on Hold Now': Migrants' Experiences of Waiting and Immobility During the COVID-19 Pandemic." *Social & Cultural Geography* 24, no. 10 (2023): 1846–62.

Hennekam, Sophie, Jamie Ladge, and Yuliya Shymko. "From Zero to Hero: An Exploratory Study Examining Sudden Hero Status Among Nonphysician Health Care Workers During the COVID-19 Pandemic." *Journal of Applied Psychology* 105, no. 10 (2020): 1088–100. https://doi.org/10.1037/apl0000832.

Keen, Suzanne. "Strategic Empathizing: Techniques of Bounded, Ambassadorial, and Broadcast Narrative Empathy." *Deutsche Vierteljahrsschrift für Literaturwissenschaft und Geistesgeschichte* 82, no. 3 (2008): 477–93. https://doi.org/10.1007/BF03374712.

Martínez García, Ana Belén. "Memories of War and the COVID-19 Crisis in Spain." *Human Arenas* 4 (2021): 366–78. https://doi.org/10.1007/s42087-020-00145-3.

Puig de la Bellacasa, Maria. "Matters of Care in Technoscience: Assembling Neglected Things." *Social Studies of Science* 41, no. 1 (2011): 85–106.

Puig de la Bellacasa, María. *Matters of Care: Speculative Ethics in More than Human Worlds*. Minneapolis: University of Minnesota Press, 2017.

Ryan, J. Michael, and Serena Nanda. *COVID-19: Social Inequalities and Human Possibilities*. Abingdon: Routledge, 2022.

Salazar, Noel B. "Immobility: The Relational and Experiential Qualities of an Ambiguous Concept." *Transfers* 11, no. 3 (2021): 3–21.

Smith, Sidonie, and Julia Watson. *Reading Autobiography Now: An Updated Guide for Interpreting Life Narratives*, 3rd ed. Minneapolis: University of Minnesota Press, 2024.

9

BEING THE COMIC ART

Loss, Creation, and Lessons Drawn From COVID-19

Christopher J. Gilbert

I had once again let my habit of drawing go by the time Kairos died.

It was early January in 2024, nearly four years after those unforgettable, mandatory stay-at-home orders. My kids were 3 and 5. In that springtime of their childlike innocence, a moment of shutdowns and lockdowns, an onset of pandemic times, the era of COVID-19, they were as blissful about more daytime hours to play as our two senior cats—Kairos and Norah—were about the new reality of their people being always around.

We were living in Melrose, Massachusetts then, in a colonial-style home built in 1900 with not a whole lot of space but a serviceable backyard. My wife built a garden back there. With the help of my dad, I built a play structure for the kids, complete with a two-level fort and a swing set. I built them a climbing dome, too. And a sandbox. There was also enough grass for them to run around in, and enough curiosity and mischievousness in their young hearts and minds for them to sneak over the fence, once, and explore the outskirts of the conservation lands that abutted our property. "Hi, Dad!" they both exclaimed from atop a steep hill when they heard me calling their names, surely picking up on the panic I felt, not knowing where they had gone. I sighed when I saw them (and smiled later with my wife when we shared our mutual respect for their industriousness in using an upside-down trashcan as a platform for helping each other up, over, and out). They giggled and grinned. My wife and I lamented what now seemed so unsafe. Spaces beyond the borders of our property. Other people. Nature.

When Kairos died, the world had mostly moved on. We weren't wearing masks everywhere we went, yet we were still wary of uncovered noses and mouths. We kept things close to home even though we were back to gathering in the same air with friends and family. And we found ourselves in the right headspaces at the right time to pick up and move to a 12-acre farmstead in northern Connecticut. It

DOI: 10.4324/9781003735595-13

was early 2022. We brought a small flock of chickens, and then enlarged it. We got some rabbits. With my dad's guidance, I learned to do some rudimentary construction and electrical work in the course of remodeling a large chicken coop, creating bays on the ground floor of a three-story barn, and wiring up outbuildings. I took to cutting and chopping wood, creating a trail system, doing small engine maintenance, operating a tractor, and on and on. Now, we have goats and two livestock guardian dogs and a strong connection to the land and animals in our care. Now, I am back in my routines of teaching and writing. Now, when the sun shines bright on a spring day, I am not riding my bike on a stationary trainer in the backyard; or playing the role of professor while co-parenting; or capturing my children's milestones and cherishing family memories as if I am making concessions; or, in the end, imagining that daily existence is a strange mix of utter proximity to the extraordinarily mundane and that reality can only be experienced at a distance. Now, when I remember how drawing became something of a vocation, how I came to drawing in the first place, I think of Jacques Derrida's reflections on crafting expressions without replies, on finding the self in something (or someone) other than the self, and even more on how my cat—like my drawing habit, like that moment from which both discontentment and contentment sprang—seems like a pastime. "(im)c-a-t(mo)" and all that about what the cat did, as E. E. Cummings once poetized.

As with a cat, so with art . . .

away
wanders:exact ly;as
if
not
hing had, ever happ ene
D[1]

So, it did not surprise me when the first impulse I felt after Kairos passed was the impulse to put something into writing, almost poetically, with no reader in mind other than me, and with no motive beyond naked, immediate abreaction. Here is what I wrote.

A light snow fell overnight. A dusting, really.

I woke up with weak eyes. Can't remember the last time I cried.

As the snow melted on the rooftop of the Highlander on the way to drop the kiddos off at school, streams of water flowed down the windshield. They looked like tears. I flicked on the wipers and wiped them away. They came back. When I parked the car in front of the barn, I let the remaining streams flow.

His name was Kairos. In ancient Greek, the word καιρός, or *kairós*, means opportune moment—the right place at the right time. That is how he came to me in the spring of 2009. It was time for him to go. He had declined, physically,

> over the last year. It was the right time. I told him so as he drew his last breaths beside the boiler. "It's okay," I said. "You can go." He didn't try to hide. I didn't want to leave. There was no hiding. Only leaving.
>
> There is a haze in the sky now. Sun mixed with clouds mixed with the general *mise-en- scène* of winter. And there is snow in the forecast. Time to clean up after him one last time. Time to do the work of remembering. Time to move on. Time to be ready, again. A snowstorm looms. Between 4 and 8 inches in the forecast. The word καιρός also means season, or fitting time. To everything there is a season. A time to die. A time to weep. A time to laugh. A time to mourn. A time to dig a hole before the ground freezes.

That was on January 4. The day before, when I could not stop thinking about whether or not my 14-year-old cat was dead in the basement . . . .

> He must be on his ninth life—Kairos. I found him restful but clearly in decline on his blanket beside the washing machine. I knelt beside him for a while. Ran my fingers along his back and through the soft but matted fur on his head. He purred, and his diminutive, skeletal frame seemed to quiver. Still, he snuggled into my fingers, leaned against my hand. "My boy," I said, quietly. "My boy."
>
> Impossible not to juxtapose this moment to the new day of cat life in the barn. The two kittens in the hayloft, Starlight and Buttons, greeted me at the door as they always do now, nuzzled and nudged for attention, rolled around on the wooden floorboards, and sent reverberations of friskiness and feline spirit resounding through the walls as I finished morning chores and headed back to the family room to stoke the fire.

And the day after . . . .

> Mornings, now, are mornings of absent presence. And this absence, this presence, will carry through the day into the evening hours and long after the next sun sets and a new one rises. He no longer needs me to serve him his wet food twice a day and keep his dry food topped off. He no longer needs me to get rid of his refuse. He no longer needs a snuggle, head to head, cheek to nose. He no longer needs to purr. He no longer needs to run full speed in that apartment on Elmbury Court, leap from somewhere in the middle of the hallway, and slam into our bedroom door. That weekend wake-up call. That plea for food and attention, while Norah sat quietly on the floor. He no longer needs to scratch at that door. He no longer needs to eat. He no longer needs to sleep. This morning I swore I heard him meow for breakfast. I swore I heard the soft scrape of his nails as he walked, tenderly, uncertainly, to lay himself down on the rug right in front of the kitchen sink where I was doing my morning work. I struggled against routine. Kid lunches were packed. Kids were fed. Erin's egg sandwich was ready and waiting for her. I had eaten. It was time to go to the basement with

Kai, spoon some Friskies into his bowl, add some raw coated kibble to the other bowl, check the water in his dispenser, freshen up his litter box. These chores. I knew it would be this way, eventually. These chores. "During the morning chores," Stephen King writes in *Wolves of the Calla*, "you look forward with love, during the evening ones, you look back with nostalgia." These burdens of animal care. These tiny joys of living and working together to survive. These lost rituals. To grieve: like being homesick at home.

This is familiar terrain for me. In fact, it represents a custom of journaling that I began and kept up during my post-tenure sabbatical. What did surprise me, though, was the other urge I felt—an urge to draw. Perhaps it was because I wanted so much to remember Kairos when he was hale and hearty. To remember him in his prime. To remember him alive. To recreate him, there, in that time and space. It was a quick sketch I drew (Figure 9.1). Kairos. Perched on the pedestal of a scratching post, in our two-bedroom, second-floor apartment on Elmbury Court in Indianapolis. I can still picture it. I pictured it. I pictured Kairos, without the pedestal.

Later that same day, my daughter saw me crying over the kitchen sink. I was weeping for Kairos. Uncontrollably. It was so strange. Generally, I am not a crier. My daughter came over and gave me a hug. Then she went into the family room and drew a picture for me. It pictured me, my wife, my son, and her, all in a line holding hands, and standing alongside three different renditions of my cat. The renditions, depicting Kairos in various positions, appeared in a circle. That circle was positioned right next to me. Another rendition of Kairos was perched on my head. "I can tell he is on your mind," my daughter said when she returned to show me what she had drawn.

What did Derrida say about first and second narratives? About acts, and creations, and *re*creations? Art captures what it cannot hold onto, keeps what it cannot keep, appeals to the want of something elapsed in the here and now. We make demands of it. It makes demands of us. I smiled at my daughter. "I guess art imitates life," I said. "Huh?" We hugged. I showed her my drawing of Kairos. She smiled and reminded me that, once upon a time, I drew a lot. It wasn't that long ago. "Remember how much we drew during the pandemic?" she asked. I did. I also remembered what E. E. Cummings said about art in "The Agony of the Artist (With a Capital A)": "Art is not something which may or may not be acquired; it is something which you are not or which you are."[2]

You are an artist. I tell my kids all the time. This was my refrain to them during those lockdowns. They both love to draw, to create. Once upon a time, I imagined myself a young artist, a young poet, simply ripening (as Rainer Maria Rilke might say) and not reckoning or counting.[2] To picture my drawings from those pandemic times is to reimagine them as the results "of having gone through an experience" to the point of having nowhere else to go but "the more private, the more personal, the more singular."[3] To picture when and where that earlier, COVID- era impulse to picture re-emerged, particularly for one whose scholarly oeuvre is principally

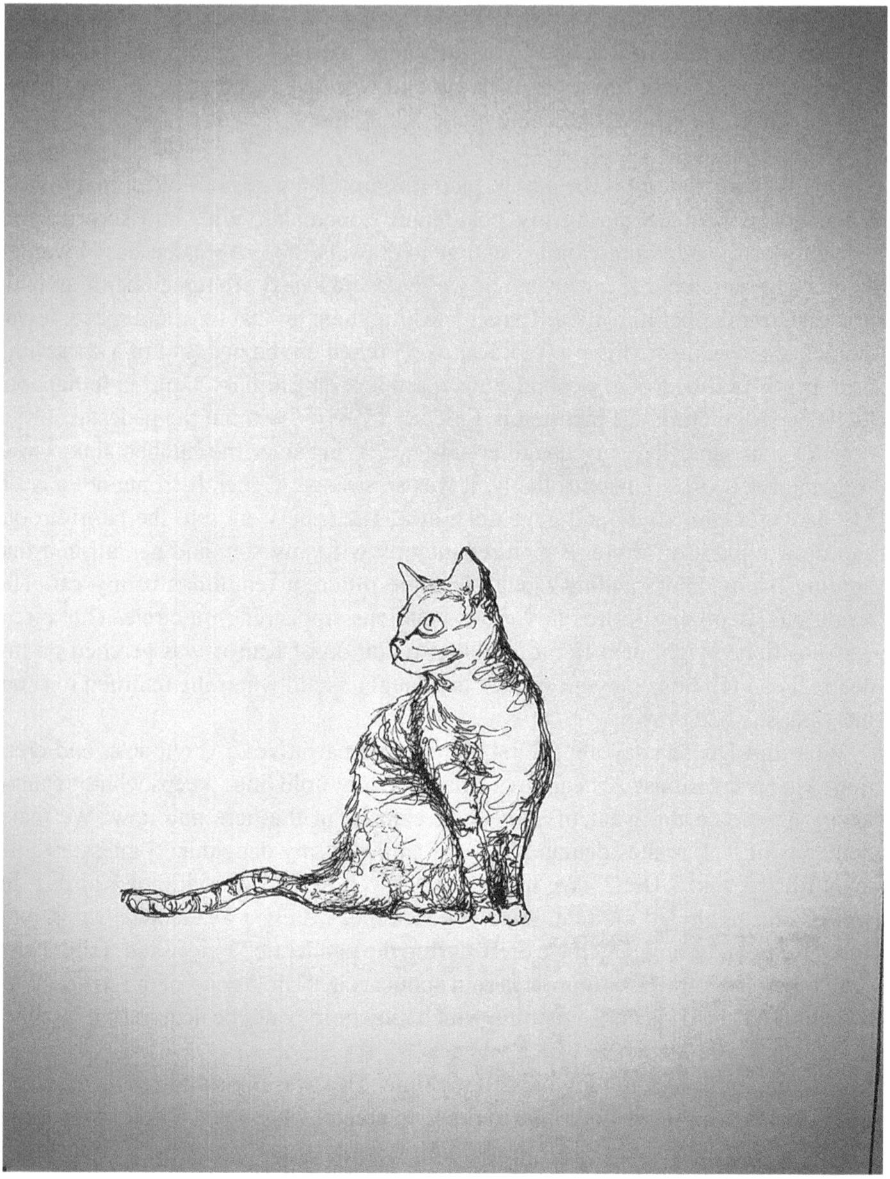

FIGURE 9.1 Christopher J. Gilbert. Sketch of Kairos, 4 January 2024.

animated by the study of comic images and political caricatures and editorial cartoons and visual rhetoric, is to reconsider not only my impetus to make art; it is also to encounter impressions I have of myself as a scholar of a certain artfulness who also deals with his own experiences in artistic terms. To picture the roots and results of that impulse, particularly in the contexts of so many new normals: provisionally, that is the task of this essay.

Unfinished Projects

It probably makes sense to assert, or perhaps admit, from the outset that I rarely finish drawings. The number of times my wife has asked me, "Are you actually going to finish that drawing?" upon my display of this or that sketch I have done over the years. . . . She is not meaning to be snarky. Quite the contrary. She champions my art. When we moved to the farmstead, one of the first things she did was transfer the few pieces of art I *have* finished (and that have been framed) from what were places of prominence at the old home to new places of prominence. Beyond those, I have countless notebooks full of unfinished projects. I have a stash of random drawings that are either integrated into handwritten notes or incorporated as doodles in the margins of notebooks. I have a collection of pieces at various stages of (in)completion in a large portfolio. There are no doubt photos of some of my drawings from many years ago in albums on my largely inactive Facebook page. Importantly, though, all of these pieces and projects represent a core characteristic of how I take stock of what I see as the weird and wonderful peculiarities in the world around me. They encapsulate how my choices of subjects reflect (and deflect) orientations that range from deep engagement to sheer escapism. Plainly, they bespeak how what Debbora Battaglia calls a "rhetorical awareness" can comingle with an "imaginary order"[4] that motivates my own approach to self-presentation—or, better, self-*re*presentation—without a writer's familiar task of addressing a readership, a public. These are proofs of and for myself, as it were, drawn from necessity.

All of this is to say that my COVID-era art moved me to account for what it means to *see oneself* in comic art, even (or especially) one's own comic art, as if a rhetorical sensibility can animate a private way of being.

A brief departure into the world of Mo Willems is a useful setup here.

Before the pandemic hit, both of my kiddos were obsessed with Mo Willems books. The *Pigeon* series. The *Knuffle Bunny* series. The *Elephant & Piggie* series. My gosh, *Leonardo the Terrible Monster*. For my part, the *Cat the Cat* series is outstanding. Maybe I like it so much because of how it seemed to speak to my 3-year-old daughter. Or maybe it is because of the polysemy at play in the noun that doubles as the naming, never mind the lessons about making friends across differences (Figure 9.2).

When we found ourselves at home, locked down, temporarily agoraphobic, separated from that dangerous world out there, I took to managing a handful of what

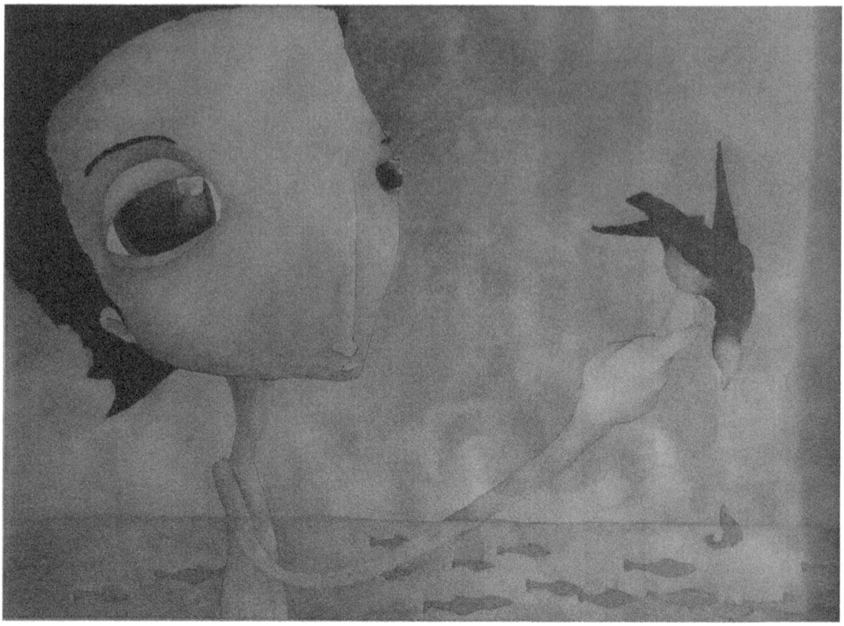

FIGURE 9.2 Christopher J. Gilbert. Man holding a red bird, pen and ink, and watercolor, 2021–2023.

had been just days before in-person classes and trying to motivate online learning while caring for those two kiddos with my wife as if parenting had become shift-work. We eventually opted for homeschooling instead of virtual schooling, and we shared the responsibility of teaching our children to do things like write the letters of the alphabet, make words and sentences, read, create and solve math problems, do all sorts of arts and crafts (like Matisse-esque cut-outs and collages, flowers made out of construction paper, and dot paintings), and generally to recognize how that little girl "laughed his joy [and] cried his grief," just as that little boy "laughed their cryings and did their dance" from spring through winter to summer and fall.[5] With his weekly "Lunch Doodles," Mo Willems became a welcome refuge.

A lunch doodle, in many ways, is exactly what it claims to be. Beginning on 16 March 2020, and running for three weeks thereafter, every weekday Mo Willems welcomed people into his home studio for a noontime activity marked by doing quick sketches, taking brief tours of his studio space, looking at some of the original dummies for his books, and hearing his answers to questions from young fans.[6] The hook was that even in isolation we do not have to be alone, namely because we remain capable of making art. All one needs is a piece of paper and a marker, or a pencil, or a crayon. One doesn't even need an idea—at least to start. A doodle with Mo Willems began with a doodle. By the end of a session, one might be ready to draw, which is to say to put marker or pencil or crayon or whatever to paper and picture an idea. The point, again, was to be—in Mo Willem's words, in that spirit so resonant of Rilke—an "art maker."

Truth be told, my wife utilized these doodles for structured fun time with the kiddos.

Occasionally I would watch. But I rarely joined in. Not for those sessions. Instead, I used them as inspiration for setting aside my own time for art. For 30 minutes, when I was "on" with the kiddos, we would be alone, together. Nine times out of ten, both children spent their 30 minutes flipping through a book. Sometimes they would build with a LEGO® or a DUPLO® set. Each and every time, I drew. I wanted to draw. I didn't doodle. I had ideas in my mind. My mind felt very much like "a big hunk of irrevocable nothing" that was being hit by "touch and taste and smell and hearing and sight," all seemingly "sharp fatal tools" working independently and all at once "in an agony of sensual chisels" that were altering me into "something a little different."[7] Such a mind can make one feel helpless. Such helplessness can be overwhelming. How does one get out of that head? No. Especially in times of perceived danger, how does one let *that helplessness* out?

In those moments of alone time, which became outlets for "sketch sessions," I created a collection of comic artworks, all blending the familiar with the strange, all representing what I might call rhetorical engagements with myself. All of the art in that collection is, by and large, unfinished. The writings and drawings that came out of my grief over Kairos have roots in these sessions, the sketches from which lay bare my "evolving subjectivity" vis-à-vis what countless artists also felt as the "malaise of everyday life."[8] They run the gamut of odd, funny, and downright bizarre. Birds wearing facemasks. A ruffled bald eagle with a torn American flag in its beak. A firefly with an Edison lightbulb for a lantern. A creepy, anthropomorphic jack-o- lantern. A bedraggled owl. And much more. What follows is a selection of some of these drawings. That selection is the basis for my reimagination of who I am (and, who I was) and what I do (and, what I did) as a writer, as a scholar, and as one who is *into*, is *in*, and, to some extent, very much *is* (his own) comic art.

When Strangeness Meets

There are no dates on any of my drawings. I cannot say for sure which was the first one I drew, never mind in what order. In the Shakespearean but also the Derridean sense, time was and is out of joint.

I also do not know precisely what first motivated my early interest in caricature. No doubt, though, that influences include *MAD* magazine, *The Simpsons*, Ralph Steadman's illustrations, Dr. Seuss's array of artworks, Etta Hulme's editorial cartoons, and eventually the artworks of Thomas Nast, N. C. Wyeth, Joe Sorren, Redmer Hoekstra, and so many other influences that stretch from my childhood to the present day.

All the same, at the crux of my fascination with comic art and occasionally making comic art myself is the notion that caricature—as a representational device defined by the exaggeration or the overstatement of specific characteristics so they appear ridiculous—captures what is there, visible, present, and yet not seen as it could or should be. To caricature is to burden or to overwhelm the ordinary with a form of strangeness that magnifies what would otherwise be confined to familiarity. A principle of caricature is precisely that the twain *shall* meet. This drawing is among the first from my sessions (Figure 9.3).

The inspiration for the impish or sprite-like faerie eludes me. What comes to mind is the fact that we were being told to mask up, even outdoors. I was no doubt riding that aforementioned bike attached to that stationary trainer on the patio in my backyard, in solitude under a warm sun, safe in ways I never thought possible from suburban streets. I was regularly going about the house quoting lines from Incubus's song, "Agoraphobia," right about the time the band released a lockdown version of it. Living life inside out. Remembering how good the world could be. Waiting in the throes.

The drawing portrays a strong albeit timorous urge to recoil even as it reflects what Derrida might dub a "strange redoubling."[9] In the act of writing, and truly the act of writing *about* something, is a wonderful, troublesome act of meaning-making. "Meaning" in writing, says Derrida, "presents itself as prerequisitely and simultaneously *read*."[10] It is no different with a drawing, once drawn.

When I look at the comic art of caricature, I do so with the critical intuition that caricature is a way of seeing. When I analyze caricature, examine it, critique it, I do so with an appreciation for its time and place, the deep history that influences it, and the everydayness and ordinariness that it expresses with regard to what *was* but nonetheless somehow *remains*, if only in seemingly bygone sentiments. When I look at this drawing, I see a caricature of what I was thinking, feeling, and doing. I see residues of a "me" that follows from the very art of *making* art as a rhetorical way of being in the world, in a form of "relation" that is likewise a "form of nonrelation," to the self and to the other.[11] I see what John Berger envisaged as the interchangeability of the one who draws and the drawing itself, appearing as the thing to be seen.

Of course, my drawings were not drawn to be seen, per se.

It was not my aim to turn them into a time capsule for pandemic times. None of them represent some a priori meaning expressed in and through an art of public communication, let alone some rhetorical act of self-construction.[12] I drew them, well, to draw. And only after the fact did each drawing appear to be "prompted by something asking to be drawn," and then betray the interchangeability of the drawer and the drawing.[13] Like this one (Figure 9.4).

Anyone familiar with Norman Rockwell will surely recognize the resemblance to his cover illustration for *The Saturday Evening Post* from February 1939. That was my inspiration, obviously. Why? I remember listening to The Beatles a lot. My daughter loved, and still loves, the song "Strawberry Fields Forever." One of my

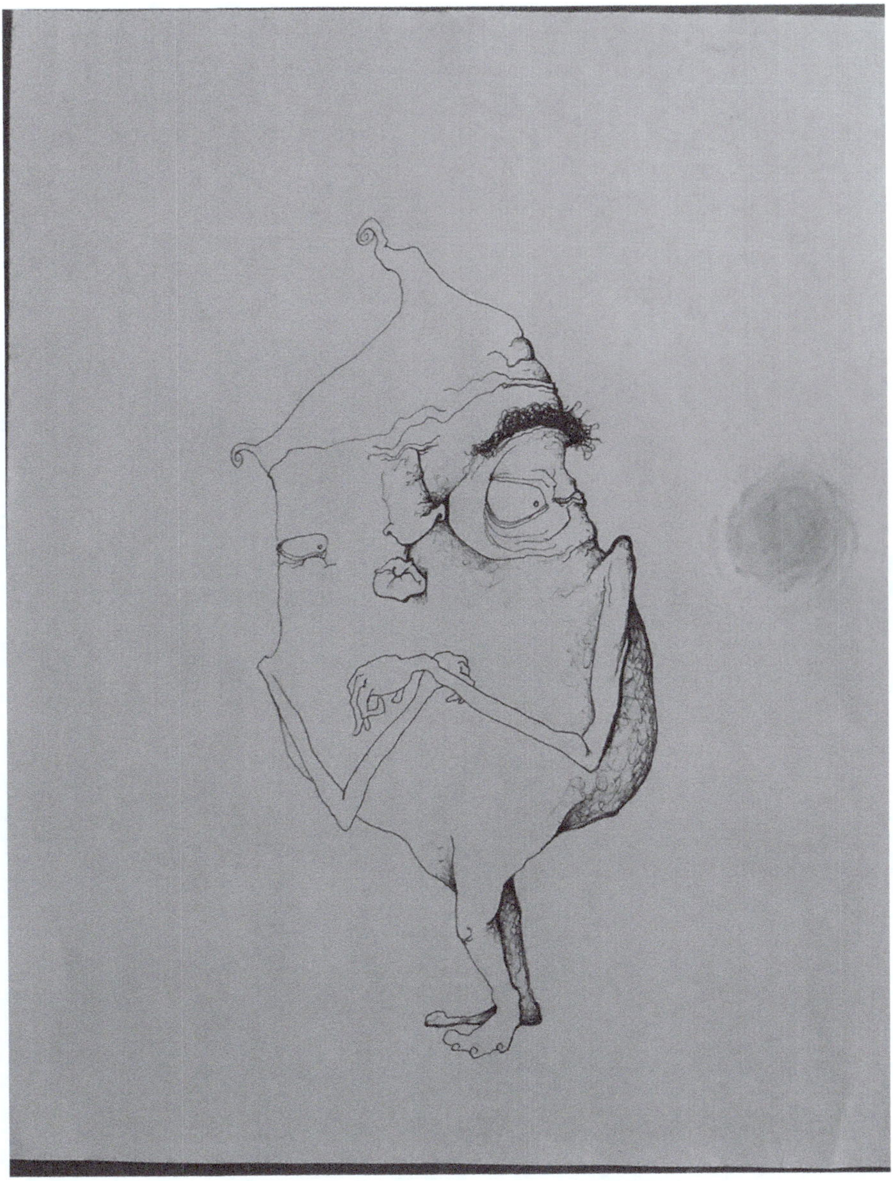

FIGURE 9.3 Christopher J. Gilbert. Drawing from sketch session, pen and ink, and colored pencil, circa April 2020.

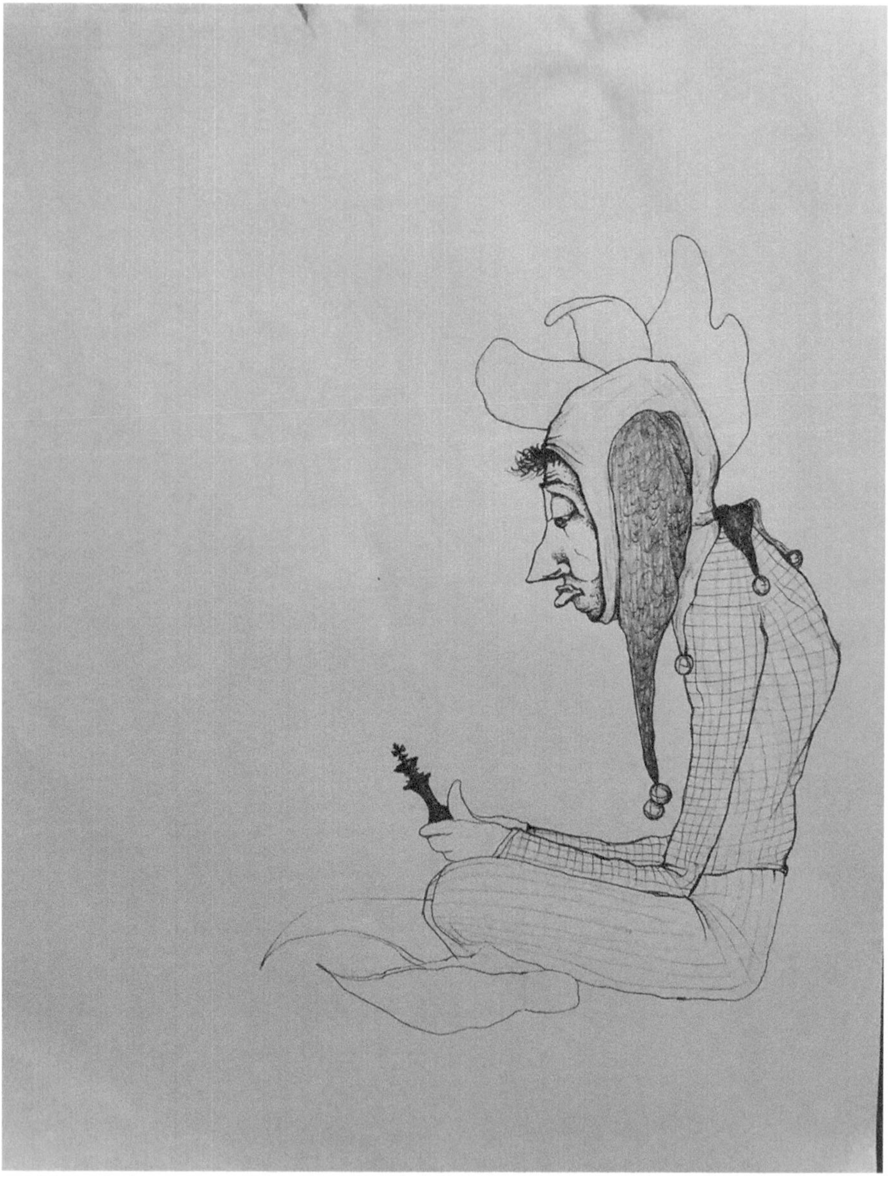

FIGURE 9.4 Christopher J. Gilbert. Drawing from sketch session, pen and ink, circa December 2020 or January 2021.

favorites is and always has been "I Am the Walrus." It's the line: "Don't you think the joker laughs at you?" I was not having a hard time finding things funny. Rather, I was having a hard time locating the funniness in reconciling inner struggles with the insecurities of the outside world, hence, the chess piece in place of the jester's marotte. It was all strategies and calculations, costs and benefits, *in situ*. Nevertheless, the cross-connections between my scholarship on wartime humor as well as historical realities are not lost on me. Most immediately, I was troubled by the war metaphors pervading public discourse urging us to fight the virus, attack it as if it was an enemy within, et cetera. At a remove, though, is the fact that Rockwell's original artwork appeared with less than two weeks on either side of Adolf Hitler speechifying before Reichstag delegates at the Kroll Opera House and Nazi storm troopers lining the aisles in Madison Square Garden at a rally of American fascists. What to do with these confluences of thoughts and feelings? What to do with the concerns about visiting friends or family members (or not), being in the proximity of others, never mind embodying a comic way of being like Stańczyk in Jan Matejko's famous nineteenth- century painting, or like a Noël Coward character smiling in the face of danger with a sort of dim wit that allows for mirth and laughter in even the most troublesome times? When lockdowns and stay-at-home orders came to be, I was in the middle of teaching an upper-level course on US American humor. I wrapped up that course in the midst of a new zeitgeist, realizing then and reflecting only later how much it really is that "a single chess piece only makes sense in the context of the other pieces on the board," and therefore any singular unit "achieves meaning in relation to all the other units within a system."[14] So much to be said and written and drawn, in jest. So many edged rhetorical tools.

Still, there was plenty of room for sheer playfulness, as if drawing was simply something I did for myself, and "for no good reason, really."[15]

Like in this drawing of an emperor penguin as a king of the Aptenodytes (Figure 9.5). And in this drawing of a seahorse with a saddle on its back (Figure 9.6).

There are outward gazes in both, incorporating images and ideas beyond the self. There is evidence of ironic distance, as well as mocking proximity. There is a sense of humor in these drawings. Accordingly, there are good reasons for looking back on them to see myself not only as a scholar of comic art but also as something of a comic artist, as more than a scholar of that which captures an I-not-you perspective, a this-not-that, the "not possible," the "only truthful."[16] Then again, it is worth noting how my own comic judgment is predicated on distinctly human standards of judgment. The COVID-19 pandemic was in part a by-product of all too human machinations. We impose ourselves upon the world. We trick ourselves into believing we can control it. When I look at my drawings, I see moments of reckoning with the sense that our jokers laugh at us. But so, no doubt, do creatures of the nonhuman animal kingdom. So do pathogens. So does the world. The neoteny in many of the drawings points toward a childlike impetus to let art be for the sake of being, and in it a playfulness that makes a mockery of its own innocence to protect attempts to defend domestic spaces against the intrusions of an outside world that

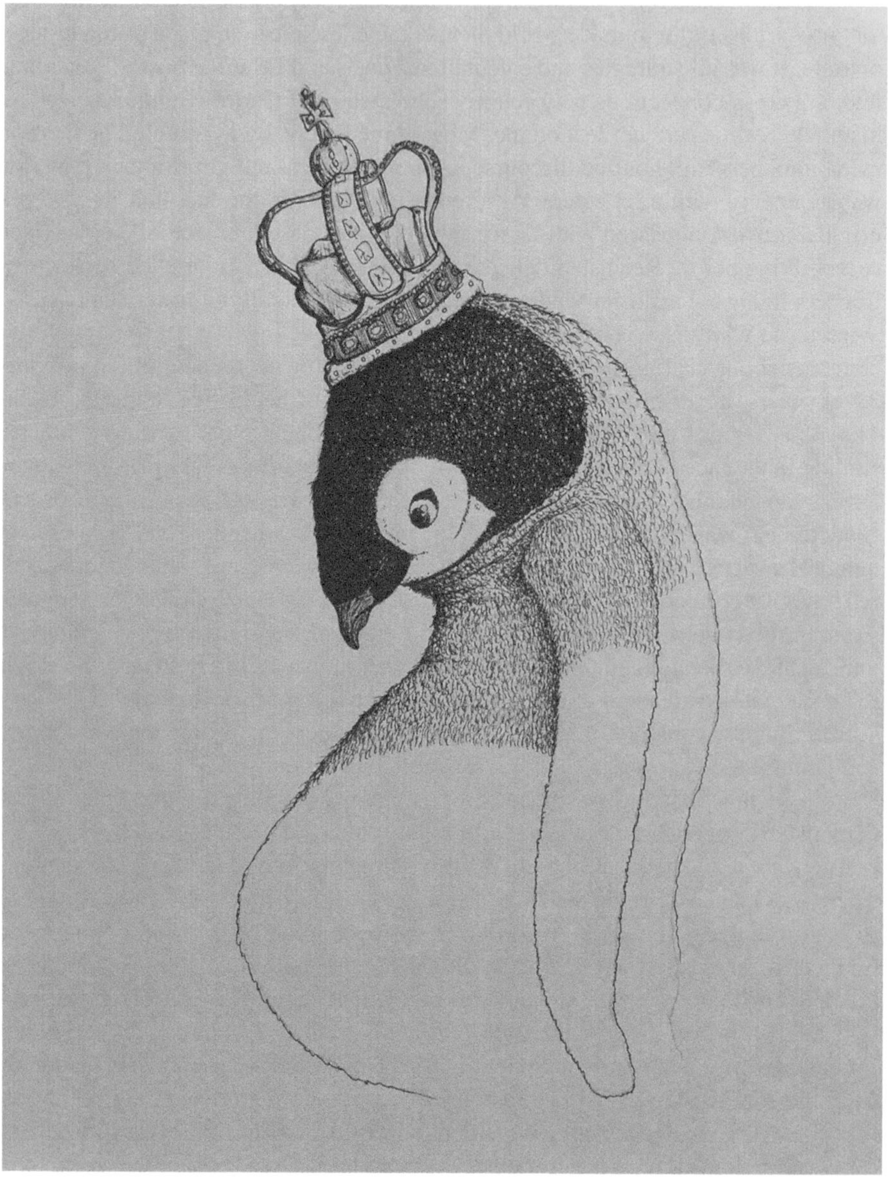

FIGURE 9.5 Christopher J. Gilbert. Sketch of penguin with crown, pen, and ink, circa February 2021.

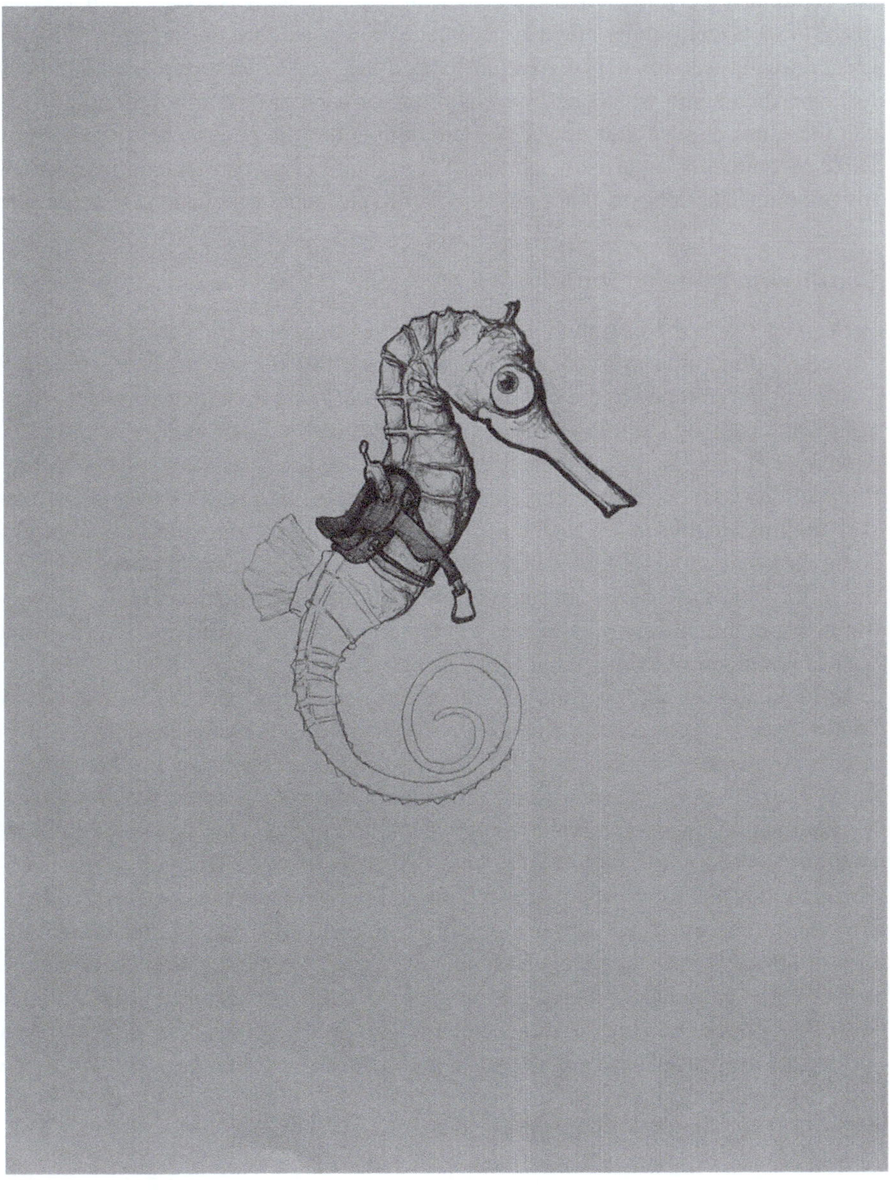

FIGURE 9.6 Christopher J. Gilbert. Drawing from sketch session, pen, and ink, circa April 2021.

reflects the tragedies and farces of adults. In the very act of drawing, I drew lessons from those intrusions. Those sketch sessions could have been a coping mechanism. Art could have been my defense mechanism. Each drawing is a page from a comic diary, of sorts, coalescing into a larger image of how we "see one another."[17] In any case, drawing was my act of creation for helping me see *myself* in what had been lost, and then again what I and we could not, or cannot, or *will* not let go of. One can therefore discern that how E. E. Cummings did his poetry (never mind how Rilke recommends an artist *be* an artist) is not unlike how I oriented the poësis of my drawing. That poësis, that orientation, enlivens some conclusions to be drawn.

Conclusion: Drawing (on) the Self

Perhaps it "is not so strange," says Battaglia, that odd currencies inform the "diversely inhabited worlds" we live in, especially during "insecure times."[18] While not in reference to the self as such, this sentiment nonetheless reflects Battaglia's anthropological framework for grasping "the nonsteady state of selfhood."[19] Moreover, it exposes the tensions between rhetorical action as those means of communication (and their outcomes, their consequences) that lead us to imagine that certain things matter in the world, some more than others, some things immensely, some things not at all.[20] And it exposes "rhetorical *self-* action," or things done *for* the self, for *the sake* of the self, maybe even for the simple sake of doing.[21] Sometimes, we communicate what wants to be communicated, as it were. We do what wants to be done. We draw what wants to be drawn.

In looking back at my COVID-era sketch sessions, I realize that examining comic modes of visualizing rhetoric (and performing a rhetorical act, visually) entails an element of examining this very process as it exists in and around any *objet d'art comique*. Such a realization reminds me of another anthropologist, Michael Taussig, who distinguishes between the "self" and the "observing self."[22] Both are more or less rhetorical effects, which is to say effects of communication activities that establish images and ideas for reconciling ourselves with others. However, to be a self who observes reality with an eye for making meaning in the face of already-made meanings is to inhabit "a world-centered and not [merely] a self-centered approach to viewing, such that the self becomes part of that which is seen."[23] Writing. Drawing. Writing about drawing(s). Drawing about what has been written, so to speak. These are all part of the rhetorical arts that might otherwise be seen as separate from any "I" or "you" or "they" or "them" who is putting things into words or picturing things, and never more so than when times are dire, dark, or dangerous—or, it must be admitted, mundane.

Back, then, to Mo Willems. It occurs to me now that any time he did a lunch doodle, Mo Willems did two things that I almost never do: first, he specified the date; and two, he signed his name on whatever he doodled or drew. He did this as an act of attribution, for sure. But he also did it to make his mark—to signify, on one hand, that he pictured whatever was on the page and, on the other, that what the picture pictured was in part who he was in that particular present, what he was thinking or feeling, and how a lived reality might be carried over into a later moment. The self here is the very self that Derrida saw coming across as if in a "strange mirror that reflects but also displaces and distorts," and therefore as an "image [that] *supervenes* upon reality."[24] In his very first episode of "Lunch Doodles," Mo Willems used markers to make a picture of a many-legged creature (and this after doodling one person-like creature with a speech bubble, "Monday," next to another person-like creature with a speech bubble, "March," and a small bird tweeting "16"). Then he wrote "MO" in the bottom right corner, an "important thing," he said, insofar as it lets people know that he did it.

I have long felt that caricature is such a compelling form of comic art because of how it holds a motley mixture of images and ideas in opposition, at once. I have also long followed Michèle Hannoosh in her sense that caricature is a "comic mirror" par excellence when it is an "agent of transformation from self-ignorance to self-knowledge, and further, to knowledge beyond the self." Examine caricatures, draw them, and one can discover "a self with the capacity to see itself as other."[25] An important thing. Hannoosh is a kindred spirit to Mikhail Bakhtin in this regard. After all, Bakhtin was as interested in comic principles as in what he variously called "self-accounting" in art, expressions of "self-experience" (and "self-experiencing"), and "the otherness of the self" as an "act of creation."[26] Art, for Bakhtin, is a rhetorical act of seeing as it is created "in relation to its material."[27] I see my drawings in this light, and in so doing I see them as drawing on my experiences of loss, of worry, and of frustration. I see my engagements with the rhetorical effects of certain realities. I therefore see them as representations of "self- rhetoric."[28] When the self becomes the material, that is when the art can be seen as self- rhetorical.

The COVID-era compelled a great many of us to live with and within ourselves, differently. Under "normal" circumstances, we are not quite so distanced from others. Under "normal" circumstances, we are not quite so close to certain others, nor to ourselves. I write this and I recall something I read early in my scholarly career, when I was first getting into editorial cartoons. Look at a "realistic drawing of a face" and you will normally "see it as the face of *another*," says Scott McCloud. "But when you enter the world of the *cartoon*, you see yourself."[29,30] Indeed.

A coronavirus world drove me to enter the cartoon world anew. Therein, I looked back at my examinations of comic art. I made comic art. I see my drawings, and draw on those examinations now, and I observe much more than a grotesque faerie shrinking away from the glare, or a vexed jester, or—lately—a cat on my head. I see connections and disconnections between who I was in writing or drawing and what was written or drawn. I see the conundrums of comic judgment. I see the world as it was and as, stubbornly, it is in so many ways, again. I see I and not-I. I see myself.

Notes

1 E.E. Cummings, "('(im)c-a-t(mo).')," *Poetry Foundation*, July 1949, https://www.poetryfoundation.org/poetrymagazine/browse?volume=74&issue=4&page=5.
2 E.E. Cummings, "The Agony of the Artist (With a Capital A)," *Vanity Fair*, April 1927, 98.
3 Rainer Maria Rilke, *Letters to a Young Poet*, trans. Reginald Snell (Garden City: Ixia Press, 2021), 13.
4 Rainer Maria Rilke, "Paris VI°, 29, Rue Cassette, Monday, 24 June 1907," in *Letter Letters on Cézanne*, trans. Joel Agee (New York: North Point Press, 2002), 4.
5 Debbora Battaglia, *Rhetorics of Self-Making*, ed. Debbora Battaglia, reprint 2019 (Berkeley, CA: University of California Press, 2023), 2, https://doi.org/10.1525/9780520915251.
6 E.E. Cummings, "Anyone Lived in a Pretty How Town," *Poetry Foundation*, August 1940, https://www.poetryfoundation.org/poetrymagazine/poems/22653/anyone-lived-in-a-pretty-how-town.
7 That year, Mo Willems was meant to be the Artist in Residence at the Kennedy Center. On the occasion of the one-year anniversary, he reflected on the purpose of his Lunch Doodles: "to doodle, reflect on a year of the Covid reality, and create abstract art together," which in hindsight was the purpose all along. See "LUNCH DOODLES with Mo Willems!" The Kennedy Center, https://www.kennedy-center.org/education/mo-willems/lunch-doodles/.
8 E.E. Cummings, "My Mind Is," in *E.E. Cummings Complete Poems, 1904–1962*, ed. George J. Firmage (New York: Liveright, 1973), 97.
9 Irene Gammel and Jason Wang, "Introduction," in *Creative Resilience and COVID-19: Figuring the Everyday in a* Pandemic, ed. Irene Gammel and Jason Wang (New York: Routledge, 2022), 2, 5.
10 Jacques Derrida, *Writing and Difference*, trans. Alan Bass (University of Chicago Press, 1978), 11.
11 Derrida, *Writing and Difference*, 11.
12 Derrida, *Writing and Difference*, 268. See also Thomas W. Benson, "Rhetoric as a Way of Being," in *American Rhetoric: Context and Criticism*, ed. Thomas W. Benson (Carbondale: Southern Illinois University Press, 1989), 293–322.
13 See Derrida's extension of Maurice Merleau-Ponty's take on communication in *Writing and Difference*, 11.
14 John Berger, *Bento's Sketchbook* (New York: Pantheon, 2011), 6.
15 Arthur Bradley, *Derrida's of Grammatology* (Edinburgh University Press, 2008), 30.
16 "Ralph Steadman: 'The Line Becomes More Aggressive'," *The Talks*, https://the-talks.com/interview/ralph-steadman/.
17 E.E. Cummings, "Once Like a Spark," in *E.E. Cummings Complete Poems, 1904–1962*, ed. George J. Firmage (New York: Liveright, 1973), 564.
18 Emmy Waldman, "How Drawing Can Help Us See One Another: From Graphic Medicine to Diary Comics," in *Creative Resilience and COVID-19: Figuring the Everyday in a* Pandemic, ed. Irene Gammel and Jason Wang (New York: Routledge, 2022), 121–34.
19 Debbora Battaglia, "Insider's Voices in Outerspaces," in *E.T. Culture: Anthropology in Outerspaces*, ed. Debbora Battaglia (Durham: Duke University Press, 2005), 2.
20 Debbora Battaglia, "Problematizing the Self: A Thematic Introduction," in *Rhetorics of Self-Making*, ed. Debbora Battaglia (Berkeley: University of California Press, 1995), 1.
21 I arrive at this sensibility to some degree from Thomas B. Farrell's definition of rhetoric as "the art, the fine and useful art, of making things matter." See Thomas B. Farrell, "The Weight of Rhetoric: Studies in Cultural Delirium," *Philosophy & Rhetoric* 41 (2008): 467–87.
22 Battaglia, "Problematizing the Self," 7. Emphasis added.
23 Michael Taussig, *What Color Is the Sacred?* (University of Chicago Press, 2009), 114.
24 Taussig, *What* Color, 13–14.

25 Jacques Derrida, *Dissemination*, trans. Barbara Johnson (London: Continuum, 2004), 204.
26 Michele Hannoosh, *Baudelaire and Caricature: From the Comic to an Art of Modernity* (Penn State University Press, 1992), 68.
27 These are terms used throughout Mikhail Bakhtin's early essays. See *Art and Answerability: Early Philosophical Essays by M. M. Bakhtin*, ed. Michael Holquist and Vadim Liapunov, trans. Vadim Liapunov (Austin: University of Texas Press, 1990).
28 See Mikhail Bakhtin, "Supplement: The Problem of Content, Material, and Form in Verbal Art (1924)," in *Art & Answerability*, trans. Kenneth Brostrom (Austin: University of Texas Press, 1990), 279, 294.
29 Battaglia, "Problematizing the Self," 4.
30 Scott McCloud, *Understanding Comics: The Invisible Art* (New York: HarperCollins, 1994), 36.

10

WORLDING THE POST-PANDEMIC

On Documenting, and Enduring Lockdown

Brent Luvaas

Photography as Worlding

The first few weeks of the COVID-19 pandemic I experienced as a constriction, an acute reduction of my world down to the enclosed structure of my suburban Philadelphian home (Figure 10.1). The rest of the pandemic I spent learning to live within that world. I used photography. I used writing. I might have learned to do it a little too well.

The concept of "worlding" is often credited to the philosopher Martin Heidegger. It refers to the active process through which we bring into being the world around us. The idea is simple: the world is not some inert thing, just sitting there, waiting for us to discover it. We are always already a part of it. We have no vantage point from which to view it, except right in the thick of it. Our perception of the world is itself part of the world, shaping how we engage with it and one another. The world, then, is built through our engagement with it, an ongoing practice of enfolding, encoding, distancing, and bringing near that shapes us even as we shape it.

Since Heidegger, cultural theorists have made use of the term worlding to describe everything from colonial practices of record-keeping to contemporary urban development in the global south.[1] As a cultural and visual anthropologist, I have long been interested in the camera as a tool for worlding. Anthropologists like Deborah Poole and Christopher Pinney have shown how photographs help us build our sense of self and place.[2] Photographs, they argue, represent, and make manifest, inner experiences not otherwise evident.[3] They provide a vehicle for us to "travel beyond the horizons of the everyday."[4] Photography, these anthropologists demonstrate, is not just a means of depicting what is, but for imagining and enacting what could be. It is "central to processes of worldmaking,"[5] shaping how we imagine, occupy, and evaluate the spaces in which we live, and the elsewheres that lie outside of those spaces.

DOI: 10.4324/9781003735595-14

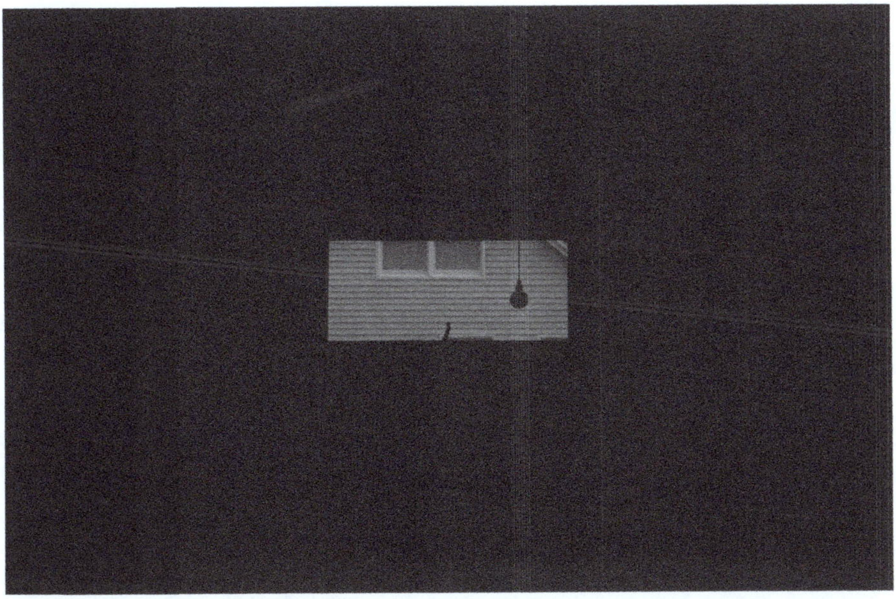

FIGURE 10.1 Brent Luvaas. Photograph of the author's home, Philadelphia, 2020.

In the decade prior to the pandemic, I studied street and fashion photography as a mode of worlding. Trained in an ethnographic tradition that emphasizes direct participation in the social phenomena we study, I was convinced that the only way to truly understand street and fashion photography was to become a street and fashion photographer myself. In 2012, I started a street style blog called Urban Fieldnotes as an instrument for studying street style blogging, the amateur practice of photographing and posting online what "regular" people are wearing on the streets. In 2016, I turned to street photography, the candid photo-documentation of everyday life in public space, as described by Colin Westerbeck and Joel Meyerowitz in *Bystander: A History of Street Photography* (1995).[6] Both genres, I discovered, help shape a photographer's perception of, and relationship with, their city. They enable them to perceive moods and trends, patterns and incongruities, what writer and photographer Teju Cole calls "echoes and agreements" that "go unseen . . . unless photography intervenes."[7]

What drew me to the genre of street photography specifically was its emphasis on ambiguity. Whereas photojournalism, documentary, and most ethnographic photography attempt to clarify a situation for their viewers, using images to provide context, exemplify theory, or illustrate points, street photography attempts to depict the fundamental unknowability of lived experience.[8] Street photographers capture the mystery of the everyday, the odd and irreconcilable, the ironic and comic. Rather than a distanced reflection, their work emerges from the immediacy of encounter. Street photography is not so much meant to be understood as to be felt and experienced. It is a practice of engagement with the affective landscapes of the urban environment, the atmospheres, and dispositions that make a place what it is. It requires its practitioners to be out in the world collaborating with it,[9] never certain of what they might come across or what to make of it when they do. To learn to do street photography, I stayed continually in motion, moving from one block to the next, one country to the next, immersing myself in the outside world, and attempting to stay open to whatever I encountered there.

And then, the pandemic happened. Street photography, as I had been practicing it, was no longer possible. In the context of social distancing, the idea of throwing myself into a series of near encounters with strangers in public was not only undesirable but also unthinkable.

Worlding Lockdown

It took me a while to figure out how to keep up my photographic practice during lockdown. It took me a while to get my bearings at all. During the first few weeks, when politicians and journalists still insisted it was a temporary measure, an emergency intervention to prevent hospitals from overflowing that would last for no more than a few weeks, my wife, my daughter and I treated lockdown like a staycation or spring cleaning, a pause in our hectic schedules, so that we could catch up on our sleep and steady ourselves for what lay ahead. We had nightly cocktails, watched whole seasons of reality TV, emptied drawers, repaired windows and doors (Figure 10.2).

But once it became clear that the world outside would remain closed to us for the foreseeable future, we started thinking that maybe it was time to build our own world inside. We adopted a rescue kitten, birthed our own sourdough starter, named it Ned. We filled our living room with an overwhelming, almost untenable number of plants (Figure 10.3). Thursdays we dubbed "ice cream night," Saturdays were "date night." Both were catered by DoorDash and an order-by-mail wine club.

We got used to the idea that our house was our everywhere.

That's the thing about worlds. They are always conditional, unstable, unfinished. We live our lives, house our houses, world our worlds. And "we"—however that is defined—are not the only ones doing this. Worlding is always a collaboration between multiple entangled actors, human and non-human,[10] living and non-living. During the pandemic, the assemblage of actors constructing my family's world both expanded and contracted.

I decided, a few weeks in, that it was time to start documenting. Not for the sake of posterity. In the slow-drag days of early lockdown, posterity was too abstract a concept to motivate me. Who cares about future generations when this one might not get through next week? I started documenting, rather, as a means of worlding, re-making the space confining me into something I could live within. If my house was a cage of beige walls and overflowing drawers, I was determined to fill

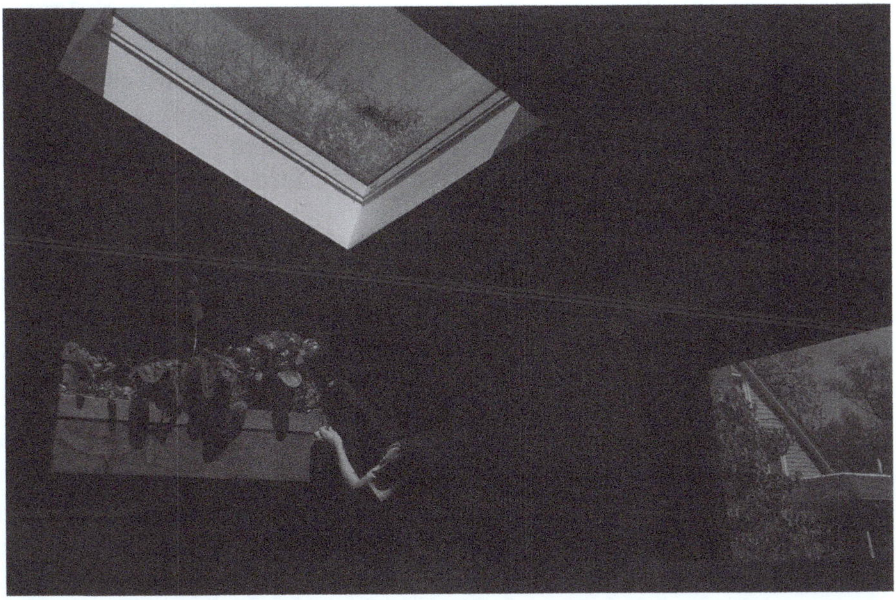

FIGURE 10.2 Brent Luvaas. Photograph of repaired windows and skylight, Philadelphia, 2020.

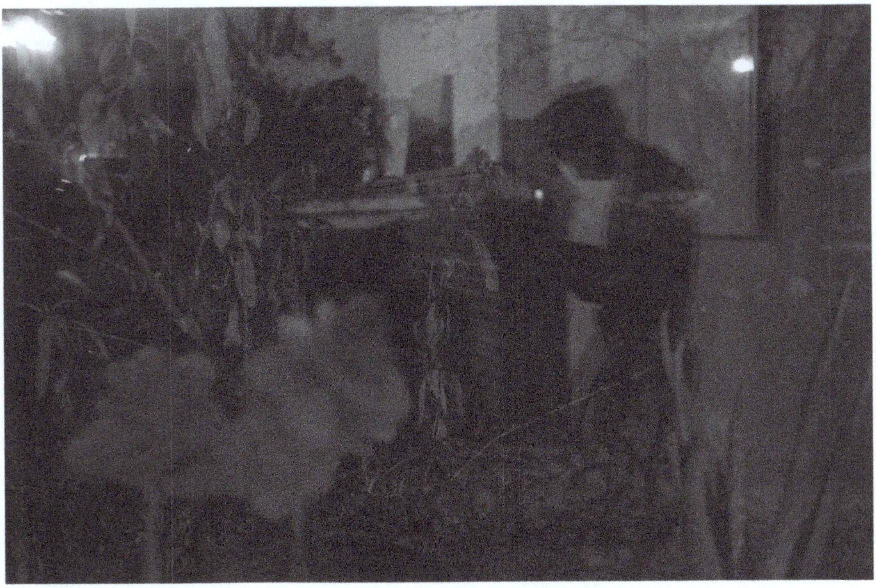

FIGURE 10.3 Brent Luvaas. Photograph of house plants, 2020.

that cage with something more. Not meaning. Meaning was for the Before Times. Something more like life. Messy. Multifarious. Brimming over.

Writing was one obvious approach to take. Since I started my first ethnographic project in Los Angeles in 2004, I have been carrying a paper notebook around with me to jot down thoughts and observations. Most of the time it sits idly in my camera bag, waiting for me to enter "the field." But when I started doing research online in 2012, the field expanded to everywhere. By the time I finished my street style blogging project in 2016, I was taking fieldnotes all the time, noting patterns and practices happening around me on a daily basis. When lockdown started, taking notes felt like second nature. My home was my new field site, lockdown my new subject.

And then, when I found myself unable to accurately describe what it felt like to live through lockdown, I pulled out my camera. I shot through our windows and hallways, up our stairwells, into our living and dining room: my daughter "attending school" on a laptop on the couch, my wife attending plants in our living room hutch, the neighborhood kids playing outside (Figure 10.4).

In the photos I took, I borrowed my emphasis on mood over meaning from street photography. I sought out the cryptic within the mundane, the strange within the familiar. My wife, herself an artist, would look over the pictures with me at night. We would discuss which ones worked and which didn't. Most didn't. There was something too flat about them. They were too straight up, too journalistic. Our daughter reading a book in bed. My wife crocheting on our bedroom floor. You look at the shots and think, "That's a girl reading a book. That's a woman crocheting."

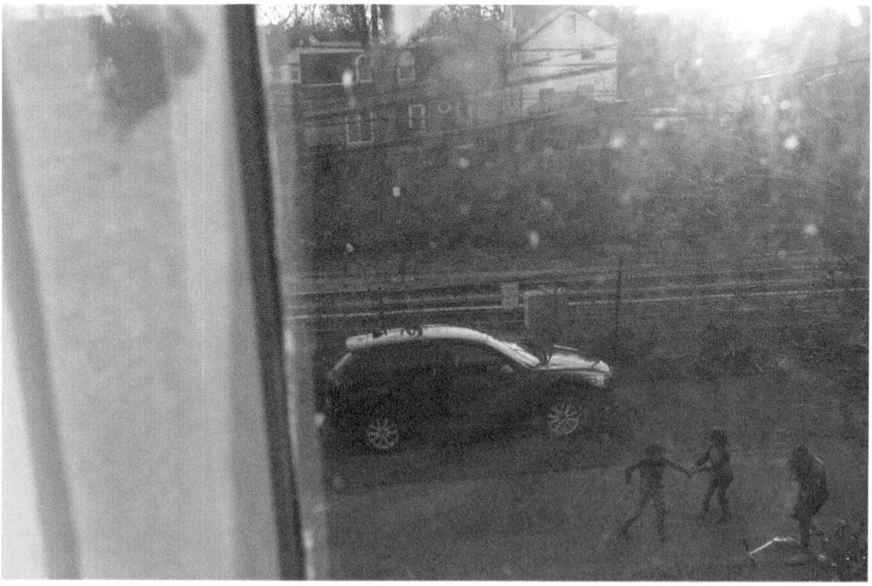

FIGURE 10.4 Brent Luvaas. Photograph of neighborhood kids, Philadelphia, 2020.

I wanted pictures that did something else. Something less clear, less definitive. That left you in an in-between space, in the thick of things, unable to pull yourself out. I wanted pictures that were post-meaning. Post-beauty. Post-world made comprehensible through analysis. I wanted a kind of semiotic paralysis. This. Just this. But this is already so thick and dense with content, you can't quite see through it.

I found comfort in that meaninglessness. What mattered was light. What mattered was shadow. Composition. A configuration of unrelated elements. Not sense or purpose. The world felt more inhabitable to me when it wasn't crammed full of signs we struggle to read. My photos helped me to see and appreciate such a world. They helped me stop longing to inhabit somewhere else.

And gradually, this world we were building through photos, through writing, through new rituals and routines, started to feel normal. Time, which had slowed to such a painful crawl during the first few weeks of the pandemic, resumed its normal forward rush.

The World We Made

First, we remade our house as our world. The top floor was my office, my lecture hall, the middle floor my daughter's fifth-grade classroom (Figure 10.5). My wife made the ground floor her workshop and teaching space. We populated the house with plants, erected temporary barriers for our kitten.

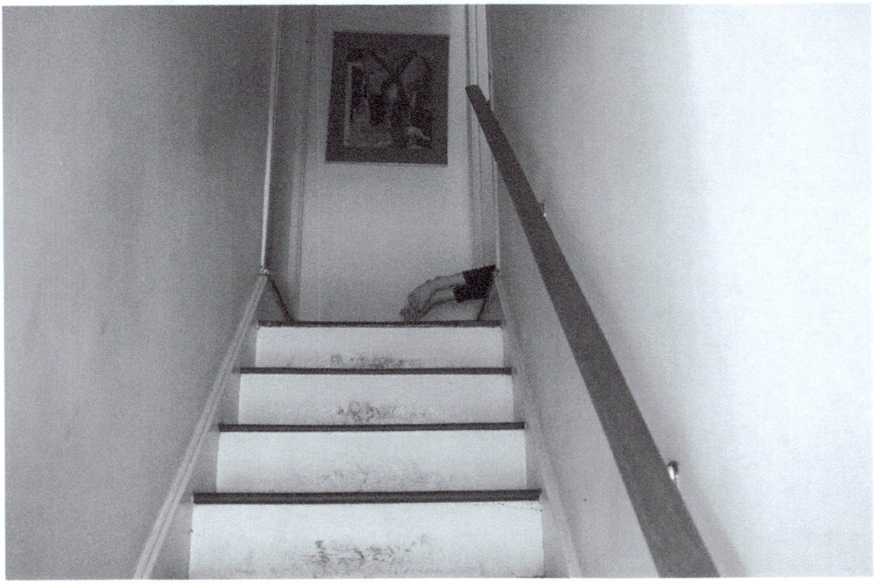

FIGURE 10.5 Brent Luvaas. Photograph of a fifth-grade classroom at home, Philadelphia, 2020.

Then, we started expanding outdoors. We took over the block. Patrolled the street. Called the cops on those ROTC bros drinking beer on the tracks in front of our house. We made the neighborhood around us our gym, jogging through its streets, taking long walks in the afternoons, avoiding our neighbors like they were the ghosts in Pac Man. When someone veered too close, we held our breaths and cursed under them. In the supermarket aisles, we shielded our faces behind glasses and masks, like those volunteer prisoners in "12 Monkeys." And we wrote about it. Took pictures of it. Gave it its own twisted variety of romance.

When my wife's father died in March 2021, we extended our domestic world still further, adding my mother-in-law to the household (Figure 10.6). She bundled up in a homemade hazmat and flew across the country with a suitcase too big for her to carry. Three adults and a teenager in a house built for two. The walls started stretching like the waistband on an old pair of sweats. The air grew staler, our breaths shallower. So, we did the trendiest, most pandemic thing we could think of and started shopping for a new house. A new, old house. A new space to fill with plants. A new neighborhood to walk through. New windows to peer into, and out of, at night.

You think, you'll never get used to this. You think, you'll never find a way to make this world your own. But you can, and you do. And when you do, your sense of dimensionality goes all out of whack, shrunk to the new reality you occupy. You

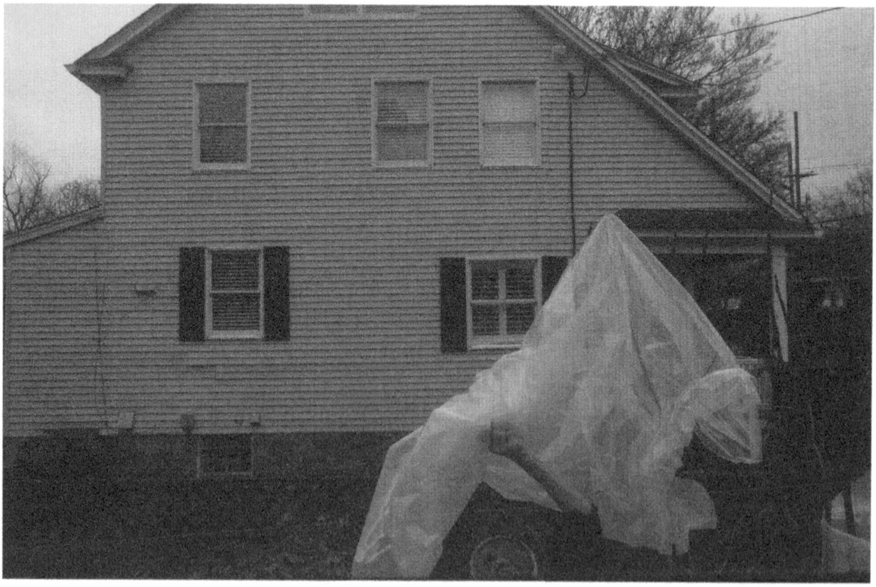

FIGURE 10.6 Brent Luvaas. Photograph of author's mother-in-law holding tarp, Philadelphia, March 2021.

get complacent. You no longer want to live in an otherwise. You no longer want to return to that world you used to know. People stand too close to you there. They spew all sorts of germs out their mouth holes.

Something in me knew I had crossed a line. The world I had helped make during the pandemic, that helped me endure the pandemic, itself endured beyond its moment of utility. I needed to do something to expand my world back.

Worlding the Post-Pandemic

I started going out on the streets again with my camera and notebook. At first, I took pictures of people only at a distance, across the street, down the block. Then, I started placing barriers between me and the subjects of my photos, literal barriers, like bus shelters and the glass entrances to the subway. In May 2022, I joined a photography workshop in Brooklyn, New York. We wore masks to discuss each other's work inside, but back out of the streets, we enacted a kind of boldness that could only be described as an act. We performed boldness until we could kinda feel some of it.

Then, a few weeks later, I went to Amsterdam for a conference. Amsterdam by then was done with masks. And social distancing. And any significant mitigation effort. People there had lost their patience for lockdown. They were ready to resume ordinary life and had decided that the best way to do that was just to do it. I was inspired. I ditched my own mask after a few days. I came back home with a few hundred pictures and a mild case of COVID.

I didn't like any of the pictures I took in Amsterdam. I was still too afraid of getting close to people, too conflicted about the ethics of the practice of taking photos without permission in this post-COVID world. And I had come to prefer the intimacy and immediacy of my pictures at home. They were of people and a place that mattered to me, subjects I knew well enough to distort effectively. My photos from lockdown held a kind of power for me that my street photos no longer could. They had forced me to look harder at the place I already was, rather than search continuously for some new scene, some new thing to happen.

Something similar occurred with my writing. During the pandemic, I wrote mostly about my own life. My emphasis as a scholar shifted from the other to the self. I was still taking notes, noting patterns and practices, but they were my own patterns, my own practices. I had switched from an ethnographic mode of research to an *autoethnographic* one.

Autoethnography is a form of "systematic sociological introspection."[11] It is a way of understanding larger social, cultural, and political trends through the way one personally experiences them. This was a useful strategy for making sense of the pandemic, but as I engaged more and more in this kind of work, other peoples' lives became more and more distant to me, more abstract. I couldn't bring myself to care about the things I had studied before: social media, street photography, fashion. They were just meaningless events happening in someone else's world.

When I got home from Amsterdam, I isolated in my room for a week, stared out the window above my bed, watched pedestrians stroll by, maskless, oblivious. I had expanded my world outward and it was contracted back again for me.

Autoethnography as Worlding

Even now, two years after Amsterdam and my first bout with COVID, my second and third boosters, my return to teaching in person, even after a series of packed theater performances, after several trips to see family in New York and California, after travel to Southeast Asia to start new research, my movements forward are tentative and erratic. I don't wear my mask anymore, but for months, it dangled from my wrist like a tired friendship bracelet.

What I have come to understand in the wake of lockdown is that it is not enough to resume our regular lives. Our regular lives aren't regular anymore. We have to *re-world* the world we once lived in, re-imagine what it is and can be, shift our perceptions toward it and our relationships with it. Aihwa Ong writes of worlding as "constitutive, spatializing, and signifying gestures that variously conjure up worlds beyond current conditions of . . . living."[12] Our current conditions are no longer tenable. We have to constitute new ones, find new ways of situating ourselves within time and space, what Kathleen Stewart calls new "form, rhythms, and refrains."[13]

I am not entirely sure how to do this. But I know that writing and photography will play a role in this autoethnographic mode I have made my dominant research instrument, and my preferred method for encountering and making sense of the world around me. Autoethnography is an increasingly common way of carrying out social scientific research. It foregrounds the felt quality of direct experience over a clear theoretical framework. It prioritizes sensation over abstraction, immediacy over distanced reflection. In this, it shares a good deal in common with street photography, as it does with other trends in life writing, particularly "autofiction."

Autofiction, writes critical theorist Anna Kornbluh, is fiction that eschews "the devices of fictification (character, plot, and narrative)."[14] Rather than creating a character, autofiction features a protagonist that shares the author's name, circumstance, and most importantly, voice. Autofiction writers transform their selves into instruments of world-building. They construct stories out of the messy, raw material of their lives. The term "fiction" does important work here. Autofiction writers don't narrate every exhaustive detail of their days. They don't simply list events or describe every felt sensation. They select. They edit. They build narrative arcs.

Even autoethnography can be described as a form of fiction, as renowned anthropologist Clifford Geertz claims.[15] It is not that ethnographers lie or make things up. It is that they construct a narrative edifice out of something vague and inchoate.

They give form, an analytic frame. Building on the postmodern critique of ethnographic writing that shook up the practice of anthropology in the 1980s, Geertz understood the generative potential of ethnography, its ability to provide structure and clarity. Ethnography, that is, is itself a practice of worlding. It shifts an author's perception of and relationship to the world around them.

Autoethnography is a world-making practice too. We can't remember and recount every detail of our lives. We can't even know our own thoughts with any claim at precision. In documenting our lives, we re-make our lives. Subtly shift our perceptions. Build new relationships. See and feel differently. Autoethnography, in short, is a form of autofiction.

Conclusion: Building Through Documenting

So, I left the pandemic as a writer of autofiction, a documenter who builds worlds through representing them. My writing and my photography provide me with a set of tools for re-engaging the world around me, and through doing so, re-shaping my sensory encounter with it.

And it's working, more or less. I can take trains now—notebook sitting on my lap, pen furiously scribbling—without thinking about all those aerosolized droplets darting toward my eyes and mouth. I can walk through crowded city streets, camera installed in a shoulder bag beside me, find moments of beauty, and hope in a Philadelphia still battered by political turmoil and economic despair.

Still, there's always some guy behind me hacking up four years' worth of accumulated gunk, testing the limits of my resolve. There's always some boarded up shop on a street full of boutiques reminding me of just what we've all lost. I can attend meetings in person now, but it's hard to resist the temptation to play a few games of solitaire beneath the table. Check my email. Open my newsfeed. Attempt to magically disappear while in plain view.

I know, however, that I have to do it. That we all have to. Re-world our world. Use the creative resources at our disposal to build through documenting. Otherwise, we stay stuck in this in-between place, where we've gotten rid of the "social" but kept the "distancing." Otherwise, we stay locked in the "auto" and forget the whole ethnography part. The other people and beings around us part, the whole massive swarm of life that is not us.

To document is to open oneself up to that swarm of life, to let it enter into you, become part of you. To document is to perceive the world differently, and to perceive the world differently is to change it into something else. Our worlds are built through our perception of them. Photography, ethnography, and life writing shape our perceptions. They are tools for making, not just representing. And making, today, is paramount.

It was a compelling world my family managed to make during lockdown, but I don't want to live there anymore.

Notes

1 Gayatri Spivak, *A Critique of Postcolonial Reason: Toward a History of the Vanishing Present* (Cambridge: Harvard University Press, 1999); AbdouMaliq Simone, "On the Worlding of African Cities," *African Studies Review* 44, no. 2 (2001): 15–41; Aihwa Ong, "Introduction: Worlding Cities, or the Art of Being Global," in *Worlding Cities: Asian Experiments and the Art of Being Global*, ed. Ananya Roy and Aihwa Ong (Malden, MA: Wiley-Blackwell, 2011), 1–26; Ananya Roy, "Urbanisms, Worlding Practices, and the Theory of Planning," *Planning Theory* 10, no. 1 (2011): 6–15.
2 Deborah Poole, *Vision, Race, and Modernity: A Visual Economy of the Andean Image World* (Princeton: Princeton University Press, 1997); Christopher Pinney, *Camera Indica: The Social Lives of Indian Photographs* (Chicago: University of Chicago Press, 1998).
3 David MacDougall, "Photo Hierarchicus: Signs and Mirrors in Indian Photography," *Visual Anthropology* 5 (1992): 103–29.
4 Karen Strassler, *Refracted Visions: Popular Photography and National Modernity in Java* (Durham: Duke University Press, 2010).
5 Zeynep Devrim Gürsel, *Image Brokers: Visualizing World News in the Age of Digital Circulation* (Oakland: University of California Press, 2016).
6 Colin Westerbeck and Joel Meyerowitz, *Bystander: A History of Street Photography* (Boston: Bulfinch Press, 1994).
7 Teju Cole, *Blind Spot* (New York: Random House, 2017).
8 For more, see Brent Luvaas, "Shadow Worlding: Chasing Light in Yogyakarta," *American Anthropologist* 124, no. 2 (2022): 399–416.
9 Alex Webb and Rebecca Norris-Webb, *On Street Photography and the Poetic Image* (New York: Aperture, 2014).
10 See Anna Lowenhaupt Tsing, *The Mushroom at the End of the World: On the Possibility of Life in Capitalist Ruins* (Princeton, NJ: Princeton University Press, 2015).
11 Carolyn Ellis, *The Ethnographic I: A Methodological Novel about Autoethnography* (Walnut Creek: Alta Mira Press, 2004), xvii.
12 Aihwa Ong, "Introduction: Worlding Cities, or the Art of Being Global," in *Worlding Cities: Asian Experiments and the Art of Being Global*, ed. Ananya Roy and Aihwa Ong (Malden, MA: Wiley-Blackwell, 2011), 1–26.
13 Kathleen Stewart, "Tactile Compositions," paper presented at the Affectives Landscapes Conference, University of Derby, 2012.
14 Anna Kornbluh, *Immediacy, or, the Style of too Late Capitalism* (London and New York: Verso, 2023), 68.
15 James Clifford and George E. Marcus, eds., *Writing Culture: The Poetics and Politics of Ethnography* (Berkeley: University of California Press, 1986).

Bibliography

Clifford, James, and George E. Marcus, eds. *Writing Culture: The Poetics and Politics of Ethnography*. Berkeley: University of California Press, 1986.
Cole, Teju. *Blind Spot*. New York: Random House, 2017.
Ellis, Carolyn. *The Ethnographic I: A Methodological Novel About Autoethnography*. Walnut Creek: Alta Mira Press, 2004.
Gürsel, Zeynep Devrim. *Image Brokers: Visualizing World News in the Age of Digital Circulation*. Oakland: University of California Press, 2016.
Heidegger, Martin. *Being and Time*. Albany, NY: SUNY Press, 2010.
Luvaas, Brent. "Shadow Worlding: Chasing Light in Yogyakarta." *American Anthropologist* 124, no. 2 (2022): 399–416.

MacDougall, David. "Photo Hierarchicus: Signs and Mirrors in Indian Photography." *Visual Anthropology* 5 (1992): 103–29.
Ong, Aihwa. "Introduction: Worlding Cities, or the Art of Being Global." In *Worlding Cities: Asian Experiments and the Art of Being Global*, edited by Ananya Roy and Aihwa Ong, 1–26. Malden, MA: Wiley-Blackwell, 2011.
Pinney, Christopher. *Camera Indica: The Social Lives of Indian Photographs*. Chicago: University of Chicago Press, 1998.
Poole, Deborah. *Vision, Race, and Modernity: A Visual Economy of the Andean Image World*. Princeton, NJ: Princeton University Press, 1997.
Roy, Ananya. "Urbanisms, Worlding Practices, and the Theory of Planning." *Planning Theory* 10, no. 1 (2011): 6–15.
Simone, AbdouMaliq. "On the Worlding of African Cities." *African Studies Review* 44, no. 2 (2001): 15–41.
Spivak, Gayatri. *A Critique of Postcolonial Reason: Toward a History of the Vanishing Present*. Cambridge: Harvard University Press, 1999.
Stewart, Kathleen. "Tactile Compositions." Paper presented at the Affectives Landscapes. Conference. University of Derby, 2012.
Strassler, Karen. *Refracted Visions: Popular Photography and National Modernity in Java*. Durham: Duke University Press, 2010.
Tsing, Anna Lowenhaupt. *The Mushroom at the End of the World: On the Possibility of Life in Capitalist Ruins*. Princeton, NJ: Princeton University Press, 2016.
Webb, Alex, and Rebecca Norris-Webb. *On Street Photography and the Poetic Image*. New York: Aperture, 2014.
Weil, Simone. *Waiting for God*. New York: HarperPerenial Modern Classics, 1951.
Westerbeck, Colin, and Joel Meyerowitz. *Bystander: A History of Street Photography*. Boston: Bulfinch Press, 1994.

CODA

I Am Here, This Is Happening: Life Writing and the Pandemic's Echoes

J. Michael Ryan

I've long believed that auto/biographical narratives often resonate more deeply than traditional academic literature. But it wasn't until COVID-19 struck my own life that I truly understood why. In October 2022, my father became gravely ill, and I flew back to the United States from Kazakhstan. I took every precaution—mask, gloves, constant vigilance. But when it became clear he wouldn't survive, I removed my mask so he could see my face. He passed away within 24 hours. I believe he waited for me. This personal experience reminded me how, in times of crisis, writing becomes not only a means of making sense of loss but also a shared practice of survival and connection.

The COVID-19 pandemic led to an explosion in writing—academic, journalistic, life writing, and all of the many varieties between and betwixt. I have personally read, written, reviewed, and/or edited thousands of pages of pandemic-related writing. As the pandemic began and lockdowns spread worldwide, many people turned to life writing—memoirs, diaries, blogs, vlogs, essays, letters, and social media posts. These writings were often done as a way to process the trauma, anxiety, and isolation brought on by the pandemic and the associated life changes meant to help curb its spread. Life writing during the pandemic became both a private act of reflection and a public form of witness, offering insight into how people coped with disruption, found meaning in uncertainty, and documented their experiences for an unknown future.

I have learned from almost everything I have read about the pandemic, but it is life writing that has most profoundly struck an emotional chord. As traditional journalism and academic writings focused on statistics, policies, and politics, life writing captured the emotional and psychological landscape of the moment. Personal testimonies detailed the anxieties of becoming infected, the grief of separation from loved ones, and the weight of loneliness. It provided a platform, much

DOI: 10.4324/9781003735595-15

like Zoom, to share experiences in a mediated way, to find (new) ways of connection, and to try to cope with the sudden onset of radical change.

As the world continues becoming digital (at least for those lucky enough to have access and know-how of such technologies), life writing too has evolved. During the pandemic (and since), blogs, vlogs, tweets, posts, and video conferences became popular, often our only way to connect and interact with others. Unlike many traditional forms of published writing, these digital expressions captured moments and feelings in real time. This instant accessibility, combined with the ever-changing landscape of lockdowns, travel restrictions, infection rates, and new variants, meant that much of the writing was chaotic, presenting process as much as product.

As the pandemic has faded from the headlines (though certainly not in terms of infection or long-standing impacts), pandemic writings have become valuable historical documents, providing a wealthy archive of moments in time detailing the roller coaster of emotional and psychological turmoil that unfolded across the timeline of a once in a lifetime (we hope) global pandemic upheaval. They provide texture to the broader story of the pandemic—details that statistics and official reports so often miss. The blog of an overworked healthcare worker, the TikTok diary of a teenager suddenly taking classes online, and a parent's handwritten letter to their child all of these reveal how ordinary people lived through extraordinary times.

The essays in this volume testify to the power of life writing during crisis—to give form to grief, to make sense of rupture, and to assert voice amid uncertainty. In this coda, I will attempt to add my own reflections on the value of life writing, what it meant, and continues to mean, to those of us who survived the pandemic, and to provide a bit of my own self-reflection on what writing meant to me as an author, editor, speaker, and human being trying to survive. In closing, I will offer some initial reflections on another life changing force that erupted during the pandemic—generative artificial intelligence (AI)—and what that might mean for the future of life writing. To conclude, I will offer what I have recently found to be a useful analogy—that of aftershocks—in understanding what all of this might mean in post-pandemic times.

Writing, Editing, and Speaking

Many have asked me how I was able to do so much work on the pandemic, and during the pandemic. One simple reason is that I, much like everyone else, was trapped. I had fewer places to go and more time to write. I am terrible in the kitchen so rather than take up bread baking, I took up an even more intense work schedule. Being trapped was one reason, but, more importantly, it is that I felt a need to do something. I am a doctor, although not of the medical variety, and so the way that I felt that I could best contribute was by bringing knowledge to light, not only by writing myself but also by helping to provide platforms through which others could share their knowledge as well.

During the pandemic I led a triple role as author, editor, and speaker, all on top of what perhaps became my most overlooked role of all, that of a human being living through the most significant global pandemic of a generation. In each of those roles, I felt a different connection to the power of life writing and the desire, nay need, to live out my sociological imagination and connect personal troubles with public issues. I would like to explore each of these dimensions in turn as I feel that each one offers a unique perspective on how to connect lived experience, with storytelling, with life writing, with attempts to bridge the personal with the public.

Shortly after the SARS-CoV-2 virus was declared a global pandemic in March 2020, I had shared a call for papers for a volume to focus on the sociology of the pandemic. The responses I got were overwhelming, not just in terms of quantity but also in terms of quality and global range. I had initially expected maybe a dozen or so submissions, presumably all from sociologists based in the United States. I was wrong. What I ended up with were nearly one hundred proposals from a broad range of social scientists—sociologists, yes, but also anthropologists, political scientists, psychologists, economists, and even epidemiologists! I realized that a narrow volume focusing on the sociology of the pandemic was the wrong approach and so, after a conversation with Routledge, the initial single volume was expanded into two and the focus grew from sociology to social science. The result of that scholarship is now the two published volumes *COVID-19: Global Pandemic, Societal Responses, Ideological Solutions*,[1] a social science perspective on analyzing the impact of the pandemic, and *COVID-19: Social Consequences and Cultural Adaptations*,[2] providing critical insight into the institutional responses and communal consequences. Those two volumes represent the work of more than 50 of the leading social scientists from across more than a dozen countries spread across five continents.

I have since co-authored a book on the pandemic (with Serena Nanda[3]), edited seven volumes on the topic, and served as the founding Series Editor of *The COVID-19 Pandemic Series*, of which this volume is part. For a long time, I kept asking myself why I devoted so much energy to editing. In most academic settings, there is little professional or financial reward for such work, so why persist? After years of reflection, the answer has become clear: because it matters.

Editing is a labor of love, an opportunity to engage with others, foster community, and build human connections. I think of contributors as a small family, and the finished product as a collaborative result—I may be waving the wand, but there is no music without the orchestra. I hope that sense of collaboration resonates not just with those who contribute but also with those who read and engage with the work.

As an author, my engagement with writing has differed from my role as an editor. Editing felt like organizing the orchestra; writing, like playing an instrument, adding my own sound to the harmony, or at times, the dissonance. Over the past five years, I have written dozens of chapters, and news articles on the pandemic, spanning academic, journalistic, and personal forms. My introductions to edited volumes often blend the journalistic and the personal, framing academic material through my own experience. I have been candid about my early skepticism and the unprecedented responses to the virus, sharing moments of regret—such as dismissing it as a "little flu"—alongside moments of pride, publishing two of the first social sciences pieces on the pandemic. In organizing these writings and volumes, I have used life writing to frame the academic, emphasizing their interconnections and mutual influence.

As a speaker during the pandemic, writing took on a new form altogether. In this case, it served as a guide to what I was going to say. Although not the shared medium of expression, writing was still essential to guide my verbal contributions. Writing, which allows time for self- reflection, was a necessary first step before I could speak, which is more spontaneous and allows less space to think.

I mentioned that perhaps the role I myself most overlooked during the last five years has been my role as someone living through the pandemic myself. Writing, editing, and speaking became as much a way of sharing knowledge as it was a way for me to cope myself. They gave me an outlet to "keep it academic" so that perhaps I wouldn't have to deal with my own personal lived experience. Working so much on the pandemic, during the pandemic, gave me an outlet and a means of understanding a world that I truly didn't on an experiential basis. Words and analysis helped me escape, engender, operationalize, and avoid, all at once, the world around me.

Personal Loss and Collective Grieving

Trauma is both individual and collective. On an individual level, we feel it. On a collective level we understand it. The intersection of the two—the individual and the collective, the feeling and the understanding—is where writing comes into play. Where individual experience meets collective memory is, almost by definition, where writing occurs. Writing is a means by which an individual can express their personal lived embodied experience to an anonymous mass of others, often with the intention that that mass accepts them as part of their collectivity. In other words, life writing allows one to both narrate their personal experience while at the same time expressing unity with a collective and, perhaps most importantly with the goals of the writer, allowing the opportunity of an unknown to feel a sense of collectivity with the author. Personal narration is where the expression of individual opens the doors to the possibilities of the collective.

This returns me to my opening—the death of my father during the pandemic, when fate had another twist: on the day of my father's funeral, my husband, my mother, and I all tested positive for COVID-19. My husband recovered quickly; I was up and down for months; my mother was hospitalized—on the same floor, with the same doctors who had just cared for my father. I had already published multiple books related to COVID-19 by that time and had been an invited speaker at events in more than a dozen countries, but this wasn't a new book or a public lecture, this was me, my life, my family. While my father didn't die of COVID-19, the virus left its imprint on every aspect of his death, and of my life.

Like many of the contributions in this volume, this experience showed me that life writing is not mere documentation—it is an act of witnessing. Grief, when written, does not resolve; it becomes legible, sometimes barely, sometimes in fragments. I share this not to center my story but to underscore what this volume does so powerfully: pandemic life writing is a form of witnessing. As in Chimamanda Ngozi Adichie's *Notes on Grief*, which open this volume, the death of a father during the pandemic becomes the ground for both private mourning and public reflection, reminding us that the personal and the collective are always entangled.

My own experience with grief and loss during the pandemic was not an isolated incident. Instead, it was a contributing voice in the choir of a common theme. Topics of isolation, grief, and loss took center stage in the life writing of many. With lockdowns in place and physical distancing the new norm even in shared spaces, billions were cut off from their usual forms of interaction. In this vacuum of contact, many turned inward, and life writing took on an increased meaning as way to feel connected, to track the passage of time and loss, and to try to hold on to some sense of meaning in a chaotic world. The performance, and sharing, of life writing offered not just a sense of catharsis but also some sense of clarity.

Perhaps the most powerful impact of life writing during the pandemic is that it offered a way for others to feel less lonely, less isolated, and less "unique." The sharing of common experiences—be it the loss of a loved one, a job, or even "just" the sense of smell—allowed individuals to feel that their struggles were not isolated. Writers recorded how relationships changed, how plans were canceled, how dreams and vacations were put on hold, and how time itself seemed to stretch and blur. These narratives offered space to mourn not just personal loss but also collective normalities. Misery loves company, and life writing served as a means to offer companionship.

Ethical Creativity and AI

As a sociologist, someone who studies society, I find it increasingly difficult to speak of hope. That said, it is important to recognize that the pandemic brought not only collective grief but also new forms of collective hope. As the editors of this volume showed in *Creative Resilience and COVID-19: Figuring the Everyday in a Pandemic* (2020), resilience became a feature of daily life.[4] Neighbors who had been strangers got to know one another, friends reconnected, families spent more time together, and many rediscovered old interests or took up new ones.

As humanity faced an unprecedented health crisis, it also came together to find unprecedented solutions. We showed that our creative capacities extend beyond destruction: alongside weapons of extinction, we developed new vaccines capable of preserving life. We glimpsed cleaner air in big cities, distant mountaintops long hidden by smog, and the small pleasure of baking a loaf of bread. The pandemic revealed the worst and the best of us, reminding many of the fragility of our lives and the depth of our need for connection.

Life writing offered a way to make that connection—to reach strangers, to better know those we already held dear. It revealed the power of words to hold presence, to resist closure. These writings did not always offer solutions or neat conclusions; they simply bore witness. To write was to say: *I am here. This is happening. It matters.*

Yet as the SARS-CoV-2 virus reshaped human relationships across the planet, another force emerged that now threatens to reshape how we narrate them: generative artificial intelligence. When ChatGPT was released in November 2022, it was immediately evident—like the virus itself—that this was not a minor innovation but a seismic shift in how humans produce and consume language.

Life writing and generative AI occupy different narrative worlds. Life writing is grounded in lived experience—it bears memory, grief, and the texture of time and place. AI produces text without embodiment. It synthesizes rather than remembers; it generates rather than expresses.

What life writing preserves—and AI cannot—is the residue of being there: the tremble of a sentence written before a funeral, the pause when a diarist doesn't know what comes next, the contradictions and the messiness of grief. These are not flaws but the essence of human writing. AI may stimulate coherence, but it cannot reproduce the emotional labor of lived narration.

As life writing evolves in a post-pandemic world, we must remain attentive to the growing influence of AI—not to reject it outright but to protect the integrity of human voice. The temptation to outsource narrative is real in a culture that prizes speed and polish. But life writing is not about polish. It is about presence.

Just as the pandemic expanded the possibilities of life writing—freeing it from traditional forms, opening new channels of connection—so too does generative AI risk flattening its power. That risk is not inevitable, but it is urgent. The ship has not yet sailed, but the dock is crowded.

Conclusion: Aftershocks

A year and a half ago I made a big move from living in Kazakhstan (where I had been during much of the pandemic) to a new life and career in Peru, the country that suffered the highest rates of infection and deaths per capita as a result of the pandemic of any country on the planet. Although still understudied, there is evidence everywhere of the long standing, yet-to-be-fully- realized impact the pandemic has had on my new home country (or anywhere else). Although I have written much about the pandemic, including the possibilities that might unfold in a "post- pandemic" world[5], it wasn't until a recent experience that I found an apt metaphor for what those might be.

At 11:35 am on the morning of June 15, Lima was struck by a 6.1 earthquake. Tremors in Peru are not at all unusual—I had gotten used to feeling, though sometimes not, small 4-something tremors—but one of the magnitude of a 6.1 had not been felt in Lima in nearly two decades. It was also my first experience with a significant quake, and one that left me quite, pardon the expression, shook up. Although traumatizing, the quake itself was short lived. The impact of the quake on me personally, however, has not been. For a solid week after the quake I couldn't sleep, feeling that every little sound, every little jitter, every little everything was the sign of another quake. I have rationalized it all in my head (the amount of time I have spent reading about earthquakes, building codes, and safety practices has bordered on the unhealthy), but I can't quite get my heart and soul to listen to what my brain (and the academic research) has to say. In short, I am dealing with the aftershocks.

Aftershocks are sometimes more powerfully felt, more destructive, and more menacing, if only because you at least have some warning that they are likely to come (there is no such luck with earthquakes themselves) and, as with many things in life, anxiety is often worse than the event itself. In many ways, many of us are still living with the aftershocks of the pandemic.

Aftershocks represent the merging of recovery from an initial trauma, time to rationalize what that shock exactly was, and sometimes grappling with our own survival amidst loss. It is a liminal space of recovery, anxiety, coming to terms, and acceptance. It is an awareness of what has happened and an acknowledgment of the possibility that it might just happen again.

Aftershocks are also why pandemic life writing continues to be important. The pandemic might officially be over, at least by the terms of international health organizations, but it still lives on in our individual and collective memories, as well as in viral form itself. For this reason, among others, it is important that pandemic life writing be kept alive. That we continue to share our experiences, our feelings, and our testimonies; that we continue to be witnesses. It is important, nay imperative, that we continue to share, to connect, and to feel.

Ultimately, life writing during the pandemic, and beyond, reminds us that history is shaped not only by presidents and kings but also by the shared reflections of everyday people. In writing their lives during the pandemic, people were not just preserving their own individual stories—they were shaping how this collective moment will be remembered. Thank you to all who have done so.

Notes

1 J. Michael Ryan, ed., *COVID-19: Volume I: Global Pandemic, Societal Responses, Ideological Solutions* (London: Routledge, 2021).
2 J. Michael Ryan, ed., *COVID-19: Volume II: Social Consequences and Cultural Adaptations* (London: Routledge, 2021).
3 Ryan, J. Michael and Serena Nanda, *COVID-19: Social Inequalities and Human Possibilities* (London: Routledge, 2022).
4 Irene Gammel and Jason Wang, *Creative Resilience and COVID-19: Figuring the Everyday in a Pandemic* (London: Routledge, 2020).
5 Ryan, J. Michael, "An Interview with J. Michael Ryan," in *Crisis and Contagion: Conversations on Capitalism and COVID-19*, ed. Ian McKay (Toronto: Between the Lines Publishing, 2023).

INDEX